CANDIDA
DIET AGAINST IT

CANDIDA
DIET AGAINST IT

Luc De Schepper M.D. Ph.D. C.A.

Dedicated to Yolanda,
Sebastian and Luc Jr.

foulsham

LONDON · NEW YORK · TORONTO · SYDNEY

foulsham
Yeovil Road, Slough, Berkshire SL1 4 JH

ISBN 0–572–01501–1

The *Coping Confidently with Candida* section of Chapter 4 (pp 106-120) was contributed by Gloria Axelrod, Ed M, a Harvard-trained communication consultant, and Mark Fowler, CMC CPA, a management consultant specialising in communication. © 1985 Mark Fowler and Gloria Axelrod.

Printed in Great Britain at St. Edmundsbury Press, Bury St. Edmunds

CONTENTS

ACKNOWLEDGEMENTS

All my patients have contributed to this book, through their questions, their concerns and positive attitudes. Some of them have stood out, either through their direct contribution, such as my dear friends Mark Fowler and Gloria Axelrod, or through their insight and intelligent questions, such as Bonnie Armstrong, Phil Gernhard, Joan Hayes, Maria Grimm, Geraldine Boyd, Diane Raiskin, Lynn Schermerhorn, Kaj Lohman, Carol Vogelman, Nancy Knupfer, Marjorie Buetell, Jan Carter, Candice Goodfellow, and many more.

Anyone afflicted by the disease of Candida should consult a nutritionally, holistically-oriented doctor. This book is not intended to be used as a self-therapy guide but, hopefully, will give some more insight, hope and a return to better health and a fulfilling life.

Luc De Schepper, Santa Monica, California

This book is intended as a general guide to the subject of Candida and is not intended to be a substitute for professional medical advice. Consult your doctor when in doubt.

Chapter 1

What is Candida?

PROFILE OF A KILLER DISEASE

In Egypt, in 1924, British Egyptologist, Hugh Evelyn-White, was among the first to enter the tomb of King Tutankhamen, shortly after its discovery in 1922 near the ruins of Luxor. Evelyn-White became one of the dozen explorers to die soon after visiting the site. "I have succumbed to a curse", he wrote in his own blood in 1924, moments before hanging himself. At the time no–one could explain his suicide nor the many other mysterious deaths of other unfortunate ones who had entered the tomb. Coming primarily to look for gold and treasures, the excavators paid no attention to the pink, grey and green patches of fungi on the chamber walls. So, in reality, King Tut's legendary curse was a really severe allergic reaction to fungi: fruits and vegetables placed in the tomb to feed the pharaoh throughout eternity, decaying over centuries, had created deadly moulds.

USA, 1985: Headlines state that a certain killer-disease has claimed the lives of five infants in a local Los Angeles hospital, while another fourteen suffering from the same problems survived. The cause of the deaths was respiratory infections, complicated by yeast infections. The children were as young as six months of age. Yet those infants could only breathe with the assistance of plastic tubes inserted into their tracheas (windpipes). The yeast organism was found to be present in the tracheas of each of the infants, while in 50 per cent of the cases, the yeast was discovered in the blood and urine of the dead babies.

USA, 1985: A 20-year old girl is in a car accident causing her severe head trauma, missing and broken teeth, multiple sprains and strains to the neck, arms and legs. Physical therapy and major dental restorative surgery, under the coverage of heavy antibiotic therapy, were routine measures taken in the hospital. However, two months later, she experienced a gradually worsening series of symptoms: increasing fatigue, feeling of spaciness, ravenous appetite and rapid weight gain. Later, she experienced attacks that were diagnosed by neurologists as complex partial seizures (drowsiness, fatigue, confusion, anxiety, crying, loss of perception and, eventually, shock). Duration and intensity varied from attack to attack. On numerous occasions she was taken to the emergency room, diagnosed as a mental case, and released without further treatment. Before coming to my office, she was confused and considered herself a hypochondriac, since she had been treated as such by most doctors. Miraculously, she was free of 'seizures' after a course of anti-yeast medication, a change of diet, and a move away from the smoggy Los Angeles area to the clearer air of the mountains.

USA, June 1986: Headlines in the *Los Angeles Times*: "Chronic Flu-like Illness, a Medical Mystery Story". S. Smith, 42, came down with the mysterious illness soon after she ran a marathon in San Francisco last year. She got better before becoming sick again this spring, forcing her to leave her job as a business manager, Running even a half mile now would "put me in bed for a day and a half", she said. Smith is among 160 residents of Lake Tahoe's North Shore who, since the winter of 1985, have been diagnosed by two local physicians as having a chronic flu-like illness in a medical puzzle that has assumed national proportions. Most of the victims are well-educated, previously healthy, more likely to be women than men, and about 40 years old (the baby boomers). Their complaints are also similar: severe fatigue, recurrent colds, and difficulties with memory and concentration. About half have enlarged lymph nodes in their necks and almost all of them have abnormal blood tests, suggesting that a common viral infection may be involved: the EBV or Epstein Barr virus. The best the two local doctors could come up with was a diagnosis: "a chronic version of the more familiar Epstein Barr virus". Many of the patients had first seen other physicians who either "didn't know what was going on" or "thought the patients were crazy". One victim recalled: "My days are pretty boring. I read or get a videocassette. I feel like a rag doll with no stuffing". In this series of patients, about 50% are as ill today as when they were first diagnosed; about 25% have symptoms that wax and wane, and about 25% feel they have recovered. Another doctor concluded that he had seen several hundred patients whom he believes have the disease. The illness exists. There is a very clear picture. The patients can't go to work or school. Their marriages break up. All aspects of life are interfered with.

Do all these stories, some harking back almost a century, have anything in common? Yes, they do! No matter how different these stories may sound, they all involve yeast infections.

Finally, a particularly frightening and sad story reached me from yet another part of the country. The girl is fifteen years old by now, but she had been suffering from colic since birth. In addition, she was plagued with continuous colds which she fought with an average of twelve courses of antibiotics per year, for the first six years of her life. Life was never normal for this poor patient. She felt tightness in the chest, dizziness, depression, a sense of inner frailty or shakiness; she had headaches, difficulty breathing and was also observed to have numerous airborne and food allergies. The school environment made her deathly ill; numerous consultations with doctors had disastrous consequences. Finally, the family moved from California to Texas, to "one of the world's most expert help centres for environmental illnesses". Aside from draining the family coffers and further deteriorating the patient's health, nothing was accomplished. The family finally moved to Colorado and rented an 'ecology house' in the middle of the woods with no roads, no gas stove, no carpets, etc.

The mother, desperate with the minimal help she received from health professionals, decided to take matters into her own hands. Rotation diet, daily exercise, vitamins and minerals, massage, touch therapy and laughter therapy brought her daughter back to a healthier status, but she still cannot leave the house . Weakness of limbs is still a problem; food intake has to be monitored carefully.

The Candida Yeast Organism

This infamous yeast or fungus does not manufacture its own food supply from the sun as plants do, but rather consumes it like animals, burning fuel foods with oxygen. These tiny microflora are everywhere, subsisting on the surface of all living things. These are the yeasts that cause the bread to rise and fruit to ferment into wine. Candida is also present on internal and external body surfaces like the skin, mucous membranes and digestive tract. It is especially present in the oesophagus causing a symptom such as food sticking in the throat with difficulty swallowing, and in the small intestine. Normally, these yeast cells live in harmony with other bacteria in a concentration of millions of bacteria versus one yeast cell. These bacteria form the normal flora of the gastro-intestinal tract and inhibit the overgrowth of yeast in normal circumstances.

The Candida Epidemic

Historically, we know of course that Candidiasis, infection with the yeast organism, has been around for centuries. Both oral and vaginal thrush were in existence over two thousand years ago. And, if we accept that scientists working in the early days of Candida research knew what they were doing, it seems unlikely that they would have been unaware of what a dreadful disease Candida was. I believe there is another reason for this: widespread Candida is a new problem. We are currently witnessing a virtual epidemic of Candidiasis. Only a few years ago the medical world viewed yeast diseases as the diseases of the future. The doctor reviewing the recent medical literature would conclude that the future is here now!

CAUSES

What have we changed in recent decades that are likely to have created such an opportune milieu for these yeast bugs? The causative factors of any disease can be reduced to four main groups: HEREDITARY FACTORS, FOOD, EMOTIONS and EXTERNAL FACTORS.

For certain diseases, the cause will overwhelmingly be one of these four, but usually all of them are involved to a certain degree. The ONE group of factors, however, that predominates in the outbreak of Candida is the external factors group.

When during the Second World War the first antibiotics like Penicillin were made available, we had made an indisputably big step forward, but things got somewhat out-of-hand after that initial period. Broad spectrum antibiotics were—and are— used for common colds so that the normal flora of the gut can be suppressed. We all know of the use of tetracyclines in the therapy for acne; low doses were, and still are, given for months at a time. Antibiotics are frequently given for the wrong reasons, or are requested by a public that insists on strong medication for a cold since they have no time (since life's constraints do not allow the time for a natural healing) to heal more naturally. The 'time is money' attitude which dictates this behaviour is not necessarily the wisest approach, as we are now discovering.

A lot of my patients tell me that the routine addition of antibiotics to the feed of chickens, cows and pigs is driving them to vegetarianism. This is not an unusual reaction. Many see little good in this practice and the potential for harm. Although people who raise cows or pigs insist that they must use antibiotics to prevent infections and promote growth, knowledgeable critics are now beginning to disagree.

Authorities in England put a stop to adding low doses of antibiotics to the feed of livestock and poultry in 1971. So did a number of other countries in Europe. The FDA recommended a similar ban in the United States in 1977. However, the US Congress qualified this by proposing that more data was needed to make certain that tetracyclines added to animal feed posed a serious threat to the nation's health.

The gravest threat is that regular feeding of antibiotics may produce more resistant bacteria and lead to their multiplication in the animal. The problem gets worse when people ingest antibiotics, thus killing off their beneficial intestinal bacteria and allowing the overgrowth of yeast cells.

Only two days of antibiotics will allow the overgrowth of Candida in a susceptible patient. And although antibiotics may be the main culprits, they are not the only ones. Many immuno-suppressant drugs and well known cancer therapies decrease the activity of the 'liver filter'. The liver, the largest organ in the body, has many functions. These include the formation of bile, carbohydrate storage, ketone formation and the control of carbohydrate metabolism. Other functions include the detoxification of many drugs and other toxins, manufacture of many plasma proteins, urea formation and many important functions in fat metabolism.

Other external factors are surgical interventions, burns, catheterisations, dialysis, diabetes mellitus, hypothyroidism, hormonal therapy ('the pill'), pregnancy and iron-deficiency anaemia. All patients in this group have an increased risk of yeast infections.

The other three factor groups—heredity, food, emotions—should not be neglected for their part in favouring an outbreak of Candida.

Hereditary factors are important; we cannot change them, of course, but we must be aware of the potential dangers we run if we neglect to protect ourselves. How many times will patients recognize that their parents went through the same symptom complex, and accepted it like victims since clear diagnosis was at that time impossible. If a person knows he risks a certain disease because the incidence is high in the family history, taking the three other factors—food, emotions and external—into account, will help him avoid that same disease.

Food plays an extremely important role in the outbreak of Candida. Yeast-containing foods are everywhere in our diet and

11

we accentuate yeast growth by the way we process foods. This diet aspect is discussed in detail in Chapter 2.

Perhaps the least considered factor is the emotional one. Emotions are part of the onset of every disease and this is becoming more and more recognized. In the case of yeast infection, it is generated by worry and obsession that gradually lead to a weakened immune system. Patients affected by Candidiasis are mostly worriers, highly analytical, calculating, perfectionist people, with a tendency to keep their feelings inward. More about the emotions is found in Chapter 4.

SPREADING MECHANISM

How does the yeast become systemic, invading almost any organ? Normally yeast cells live in harmony in our gastro-intestinal system (especially in the oesophagus, small intestine and in the faeces). They co-exist with bacteria in a concentration of millions of bacteria to one Candida. These bacteria form the normal flora of the gastro-intestinal tract and inhibit the overgrowth of the Candida. This process is called symbiosis: it is the mutual cohabitation of living organisms with benefit to both. What is this normal intestinal flora? It consists of three parts: the main flora, the accompanying and the residual flora. The main flora are anaerobic bacteria (Bacterium bifidus and Bacteroides); the secondary one consists of the E. coli, Enterococci and Lactobacilli; the residual one is composed of yeast cells, Clostridia and Staphylococci. This becomes important when we have to replace flora that has been destroyed: the supplement that contains most of these bacteria will obviously be the best, a guideline as to which brand of 'Acidophilus' to choose. We also have to keep in mind that in cases of a disturbed relationship between the body and its physiological flora, the Bacterium bifidum especially will be suppressed.

Through several causes, like the over-use of antibiotics discussed previously, the concentration of millions of bacteria versus one Candida, changes to one bacterium versus millions of Candida cells. In normal circumstances, Candida cells do not leave the gastro-intestinal tract and spread in the blood. However, the barrier is broken when there is a concentration of millions of yeast cells, a process called PERSORPTION. Another spreading mechanism is the invasive growth of mycelia (the 'legs' of the Candida cells) in the bowel walls so that the blood and lymph vessels can be reached. Indeed, Candida can take two forms: the yeast form, which cannot penetrate the small intestine wall, and the fungal form with its mycelia, which can invade the wall and spread to the blood.

From practical experience, we know that the disease almost always becomes systemic after 6 to 12 months. Unfortunately, because of late recognition, this is almost always the case. It is this spreading to the blood that we measure when we do blood tests, but those same lab tests will not give us any indication about the prevalence of Candida in the gastro-intestinal tract.

The organ first invaded is the liver, since the portal vein, the big vessel going to the liver, seems to be the main carrier for yeast cells. This has a detrimental effect on the detoxification capacity of the patient, since the liver is THE organ which deals with this process. From there, the yeast cells spread easily to the lungs, heart and other organs.

There is, however, a third way of spreading, as the story about the babies in the Los Angeles County hospital shows: direct infection. Infection is a real danger in intensive care and in any form of catheterisation: intravenous feeding, bladder catheters and dialysis instruments can all be the primary source of Candida. Another way of direct infection happens during surgery. In the medical literature, for instance, we find examples of mycotic (yeast) endocarditis after heart valve surgery.

How Candida is Helped to Spread

There is no doubt that we are facing an important stage in the understanding of our health maintenance. Emotions, hereditary factors, medications, food abuse and environmental laxity have left our immune systems weakened. Diseases caused by EBV, CMV (Cytomegalovirus), Herpes Simplex, Hypoglycaemia, Candidiasis, Leukaemia and AIDS have so many symptoms in common because they start from the same point on our pathway to destruction: a totally suppressed immune system. Many patients suffering from Candidiasis in the early stages of disease will die in hospitals with the diagnosis of Leukaemia or AIDS. Candidiasis is a disease which will stay around for a long time unless we are willing to make drastic changes in our lifestyle. And, it is no help that 90% of the medical profession does not recognize the syndrome or brushes the matter under the carpet by claiming it is 'a fad'. However, I am confident that we will turn the odds because I have confidence in the patients themselves. Under their pressure, we, as a medical community, will be forced to look into this issue.

If there is one good aspect about this disease, it is that we will have to change our lifestyles: patients going through the rigorous diet, the self study of their inner being, the heavy emotions they have to go through such as rejection, isolation, depression, anger and frustration, will forever stay on the right track! A disease such as Candidiasis stays with you for the rest of your life. For any Candida patient with the right attitude, it will not be too difficult to fight abuse in their diet and environment. We have no choice: we get the disease or the disease gets us!

Is Candidiasis a deadly disease? Looking at the mechanism of Candidiasis, it is clear that we get the disease because our immune system is suppressed. Once the yeast cells spread to the blood stream and the organs, our immune system reacts by forming antibodies and eventually becomes exhausted. The next step is the contraction of all kinds of viral diseases such as these caused by Cytomegalovirus (CMV) and Epstein Barr virus (EBV), or Herpes Simplex I and II. Further down the same road, people may contract leukaemia, cancer or AIDS.

Studies performed in Europe showed that gastro-intestinal X-rays—performed within 4 weeks of death were normal in 11 of 14 patients in spite of the presence of severe Candida oesophagitis. None of those patients were examined for Candidiasis because the diagnosis of gastro-intestinal Candida was never considered.

Candida is frequently found in the gastro-intestinal tract of normal people, especially elderly people who seem to harbour more fungi and less lactobacilli. Using stool cultures, we know that the pathogenic phase of gastro-intestinal Candidiasis is associated with the presence of mycelia in the stools.

As already mentioned, Candida is most frequently present in the oesophagus of the patient. Hence, an endoscopy is the best single method, at least for the orthodox doctor, for diagnosing oesophageal Candidiasis.

SYMPTOMS OF CANDIDA INFECTION

How do we recognize that we may possibly be a yeast patient or, in other words, what is the typical profile of a Candida patient? The symptomatology of Candidiasis is a doctor's delight! Don't misunderstand me. It is not because the diagnosis is easy, but because the broad pattern of symptoms gives each specialist in the medical field the opportunity to have a crack at the disease. That is exactly what happens. Patients consult their gynaecologists for vaginal yeast infection and are prescribed anti-fungal cream or vaginal tablets to take as a result. The vaginal discharge seems to disappear after 5-6 days but recurs with the next menstrual cycle or right after sexual intercourse. Again, the same or maybe another local medication is prescribed. For women who have the problem during intercourse, a low dosage is advised each time after intercourse. It is not fun any more when this repeats itself over several years, and I am sure some people could even get tired of sex when it must be followed by yet another 'pill'.

At some point in the story, either the gynaecologist or the patient gets tired of the situation and the focus will be shifted on to some other symptoms. There is a wide variety of choices here. Would we like to start with the allergic symptoms and spend time and money on all the different food tests which inevitably will show some positive result? With the amount of preservatives, hormones and antibiotics we put in our food, it takes a very robust immune system not to crumble under the pressure. At this point, we go through our first change of diet. Swiftly, we omit some ten or twenty foods from our diet, with varying results. We feel somewhat well on some days, but a lot worse on other days. But do not allow yourself to become desperate. Another allergy test a couple of months later shows some new food allergies! Again, twenty more foods are omitted from our diet and we start having problems getting our daily menu together. Not unusually it becomes impossible to eat at all, because our bodies react to any food intake. "I am allergic to everything" and "I feel best when I do not eat" are frequent complaints heard from such patients. Thirty pounds in weight and several hundred pounds in money lighter, we finally find our way to the gastro–enterologist because the bloating, gas and constipation becomes just too much for the patient (and his/her partner) to take. Tests usually show nothing but an 'irritable bowel syndrome' or 'spastic colon'. At this point, if we are lucky, some dietary advice is provided but, more likely, an anti-flatulence medication, laxative or anti-spasmodic is prescribed. What a disappointment for patient and doctor when the symptoms have a tendency to get worse. The thought that the symptoms might have something to do with our 'nerves' is then thrown into the air. This may prompt us to go on with our search for the right healer. Most Candida patients will see an ENT specialist for postnasal drip, an arthritis specialist for their muscle and joint pains, a urologist for their urinary symptoms, and the final specialist will, inevitably, be the psychiatrist!

Different specialists, fed up with the lack of results and the growing frustration of the patient, opt for the most obvious cause and the patient is told: "It is all in your head" or "You have a psychosomatic disease". Even spouses at this moment are convinced that their partners either enjoy being sick or might indeed have something wrong emotionally.

Several visits to the emergency rooms for attacks, variously diagnosed as 'hysteria', 'hypoglycaemia attacks' or 'seizures' only support the belief of the different doctors. Spouses accept it and what can the patient do at this point? Psychiatry seems to be the inevitable answer. Are we not suffering from mood swings, deep depressions, even suicidal tendencies? Memory and the ability to think seem to go up and down, while attention span has totally disappeared. I remember a patient who was a dance instructor. Standing in front of her class, she wanted to say: "Take your ankle," but she actually could not recall the word. Imagine the situation: 25 students staring at their teacher who is pointing at her ankle but cannot remember that simple word. No, it is no wonder that almost ALL Candida patients land on the couch of the psychiatrist. Most of the attention at this point, of course, will be directed towards the depression, which is severe in most cases. Rejection by everyone turned to, isolation in the family, and the loss of most friends only add to the depression at this stage. And the search for an ultimate cure becomes a long and expensive calvary: admission to a mental ward for some months and even electro shock treatment often seem a logical step at this point. I can only feel great sympathy for Candida patients at this stage. Cut away from any support and subjected to hospital food seems to give them the final push. I wonder how many depressed patients there are in mental institutions who are actually Candida patients?

In many publications you may read about medical breakthroughs and claims of new discoveries for Candida or other yeast infections. However, as in many other areas of life, we have simply been blind to the factors of Candidiasis for a very long time. All we have to do is look backwards to ancient medicines. Taking another approach allows an almost immediate diagnosis. However, that diagnosis will not necessarily have the same name—but then the name of a diagnosis has never guaranteed a good treatment. Let me prove it to you in the case of Candida. Five thousand years ago in China, a Candida patient would have been diagnosed as having an 'ENERGY-DEFICIENT SPLEEN-PANCREAS' (in Chinese medicine, both organs are considered as one).

What are the functions of the spleen? The main function of this organ is transportation and transformation of food stuffs. It is the main organ of digestion and its proper function provides good appetite and good bowel movement. Lack of energy in this organ will, therefore, show initial gastro-intestinal symptoms: bloating, abdominal distension, diarrhoea changing quickly into constipation, loss of weight, although initially there might be a difficulty in losing weight, heartburn, indigestion, bad breath and mucus in the stools. Some foods such as raw and cold ones will decrease the energy in the spleen sooner than others, but when the deficiency becomes profound, any food intake will be followed by a reaction resembling an allergic symptom to those foods. In reality, they are not; it is the spleen showing it does not have the strength to do its job.

Another major function of the spleen is the production of the blood and, especially, white blood cells. Hence its enormous importance in maintaining the immune system, since white blood cells (T cells, B cells and Helper cells) are the defenders of our body. Deficient function will impair host immune response resulting in recurrent infections.

When we look at the prevalence of the modern diseases caused by viruses such as Epstein Barr Virus (EBV), Cytomegalo-viruses (CMV), recurrent Herpes Simplex and AIDS, most of these diseases have many symptoms in common because all of them are spleen-deficient syndromes. Since the spleen produces blood for all the organs, a spleen deficiency translates into mental fatigue, drowsiness, inability to concentrate, dizziness, a drained feeling, a feeling of spaciness, poor memory and general numbness. These are all blood-deficiency symptoms.

According to acupuncture theory, the spleen not only produces the blood, but it is also responsible for keeping it in the vessels. Therefore, abnormal gum bleeding and menstrual irregularities such as intermenstrual bleeding, polymenorrhoea, heavy bleeding and hormonal imbalances (PMS and dysmenorrhoea) may come into the picture.

The role of the spleen in our fluid metabolism is manifest at different levels: at that of the intestines—causing diarrhoea—, at that of the bladder—causing anuria—and at that of the subcutaneous level, producing oedema.

There are some other interesting observations to be made on Candida patients which are easily explained through acupuncture. Every Candida patient knows that he or she will be worse on muggy, damp days, or in houses with a lot of humidity and moulds. There is also a typical craving for sweets. Five thousand years ago, the Chinese observed that there was a relationship between certain organs and climatic factors. They called these the Exterior Pernicious Factors: Cold was associated with the kidney organ, Heat with the heart, Dryness with the lung, Wind with the liver, and Dampness with the spleen. Humidity is THE enemy of the spleen, decreasing the energy in this organ dramatically. In the case of Candida, deficiency of energy in the spleen is precisely the root of the problem.

Another relationship exists between the organ and the sense of taste. To each organ belongs a taste which feeds the organic energy-deficiency if given in moderate quantities, but will decrease that same energy if consumed in high quantity. And we can almost guess it, the taste belonging to the spleen is 'sweet'. Cravings for sweets are the major sign of a spleen in distress. Artificial sweeteners, for instance, some five times sweeter than sugar, present an increased danger for this organ.

And is it not interesting that many Candida patients have been diagnosed as being hypoglycaemics? Remember what we said about the spleen-pancreas entity? In other words, hypoglycaemia is nothing else than a precursor of Candida. It makes such patients more susceptible to yeast infections. As we can see, patients with this syndrome were diagnosed 5000 years ago.

Another frequent symptom noted in the history of almost every Candida patient is cystitis: frequent urination, burning feeling and urgency. However, it is a big mistake, frequently made by the patient and the medical profession, to prescribe antibiotics before the result of the urine analysis and culture has came back. Very frequently, the result will be negative since the elimination of the Candida via the urine will mimic these symptoms. Mistakenly, routine antibiotics are frequently prescribed in these conditions. If you suffer from cystitis, you can always take cranberry juice (a natural killer of urinary bacterias), and Pyridium 200 mg, for the burning feeling. Once the results of the culture are known, if an antibiotic is necessary, at least you have the choice of the least damaging one. You can also double doses of Acidophilus to protect the gastro-intestinal flora so that yeast infections are restricted to a minimum.

Another almost constant observation is the aggravation of symptoms one week before the menstrual cycle. Another possibility is the appearance of a vaginal infection just before the cycle. How can this be explained? The progesterone level increases the week before bleeding. One of the effects of the increased progesterone is the increase of the glycaemia (glucose in the blood). This glucose, a sugar, is exactly what those yeast cells thrive on. Inevitably in this period, the yeast infection which was latent in that patient, exacerbates and becomes clinically apparent. No wonder that cravings for sugar are most prominent at this moment: the increased amount of yeast cells wants food; they are in fact screaming for food and most patients oblige. Many patients with PMS will fall into this category: the increased sugar intake will make them depressive, irritable and subject to mood swings. As we can see with those patients, neither hormonal intake nor intake of the popularly recommended vitamin B6, will improve this situation. One fact is sure: females with Candidiasis also have PMS.

Another very annoying symptom is the irritation and burning feeling of the mucosae: around the anus, the vagina, the mouth and lips, and even the mucosae of the stomach, which will create a constant hungry feeling. Again, knowledge of acupuncture will save us here: the mucosae fall under the domain of the spleen; this organ is attacked by 'Heat-Dampness'. Frequently, the patient feels 'hot' inside his body. He can easily follow this up by looking at his tongue picture, especially in the morning: a thick yellow coating in the middle of the tongue is seen. When the patient gets better, the yellow thick coating becomes thin and whitish, the most objective sign he or she can observe.

A very annoying symptom is brainfog: concentration and attention span are minimal. It seems that a Candida patient has to read everything at least three times more than anybody else, and to his or her despair, is unable to retain it. It also seems to be the symptom that disappears last: most of the symptoms have improved or disappeared before 'the curtain lifts from the brain'.

What are the causes? I think they are threefold. The first one is the formation of toxins, discussed in the section on die-off symptoms (page 89). The second, as we mentioned above, is the deficient production of blood by the spleen, providing less blood for the brain.

But there is a third one! With most Candida patients, I observe neck pain due to muscle spasms. When you say 'muscle spasms', you refer in acupuncture to excessive energy in the liver-organ. The emotions linked to this organ are anger, irritability and frustration! And, do you know of any Candida patient who has not these emotions in storage? Rejection, being laughed at, subjected to modern torture such as electro shocks, have instilled most patients with these emotions. The spasms in their turn will again decrease the flow of the posterior circulation to the brain. Acupuncture, acupressure or chiropractic adjustments will be the answer.

Is this disease contagious? Only when there are active lesions in the mouth (thrush) or in the vagina. Otherwise, there is no danger of passing this debilitating disease over to your family or friends.

But it is socially contagious! Let me explain this. Once one partner suffers from Candida, the other partner becomes almost immediately a victim. There are so many dietary restrictions; most patients become sensitive to perfumes, ink, smoke, petrol fumes, . . . that it is almost impossible for that couple to socialise. This often leads to tension, anger, frustration and rejection, all emotions that are fuel for the disease. Often the Candida patient has guilt feelings for being 'such a pest', hindering the recuperation. This disease is surely a test for the stability of any relationship. So how do we diagnose this giant killer?

A SELF-SCORING DIAGNOSTIC TEST

Fill in this easy questionnaire and you will have a fairly accurate idea if you suffer from the Candida Syndrome. If you answer at least 75% 'yes' on the following questions, yeast-connected health problems are almost certainly present.

A. PAST MEDICAL HISTORY

1 Have you had or are you suffering from diseases such as:

	YES	NO
• Hypothyroidism?	☐	☐
• Hypoglycaemia?	☑	☐
• Diabetes mellitus?	☐	☐
• Cancer in any form?	☐	☐
• Burns?	☐	☑
• Iron-deficiency anaemia?	☑	☐

2 Have you ever been subjected to:

	YES	NO
• Operations?	☑	☐
• Catheterisations?	☑	☐
• Intake of cytostatic (anti-cancer) drugs; radiation therapy?	☐	☐

3 Have you been prescribed: YES   NO
   - Antibiotics, especially broad-spectrun penicillin types?   ☑   ☐
   - Tetracyclines for treatment for acne?   ☐   ☐
   - Birth control pills?   ☑   ☐
   - Cortisone, orally in the form of injection (intra-muscular or intra-articular)?   ☐   ☐

4 Have you lived in or do you live in:
   - damp climate?   ☑   ☐
   - mouldy house?   ☑   ☐
   - near a foggy beach?   ☐   ☐

5 Have you been or are you an alcohol abuser?   ☐   ☑

Have you used or are you using marijuana, cocaine or heroin?   ☐   ☑

Do you smoke?   ☐   ☑

6 Have you had recurrent viral or bacterial infections?   ☑   ☐

7 Do you have an increased intake of raw food (eg from salad bars)?   ☐   ☑

8 Have you had recurrent yeast infections (eg vaginal or nail infections)?   ☑   ☐

B. PRESENT HISTORY

9 Are your symptoms worse:
   - when you are exposed to hay?   ☐   ☐
   - when you rake dry leaves?   ☐   ☐
   - when you are near a lawn that's being mowed?   ☐   ☐
   - when you are in a damp basement?   ☐   ☐

10 Do you have a craving for:
   - Sugar?   ☑   ☐
   - Breads?   ☑   ☐
   - Alcohol?   ☐   ☐

11 Do you feel increasingly uncomfortable YES   NO
   with your environment? (reacting to
   smoke, fumes, perfumes, pesticides,
   public places)?   ☑   ☐

12 Are you allergic to Penicillin?   ☑   ☐

C. GASTRO-INTESTINAL SYMPTOMS

Are the following symptoms present?
- Gas   ☑   ☐
- Abdominal distention   ☑   ☐
- Diarrhoea   ☑   ☐
- Constipation   ☑   ☐
- Haemorrhoids   ☑   ☐
- Abdominal pain   ☑   ☐
- Anal itching   ☐   ☐
- Mucus in stools   ☐   ☐
- Heartburn   ☐   ☐
- Indigestion   ☑   ☐
- Bad breath   ☑   ☐
- Thrush   ☑   ☐
- Constant hungry feeling   ☑   ☐
- Food allergies   ☑   ☐
- Weight loss or gain without change
  of diet   ☐   ☑
- Do you have a thick white or yellow
  fur in the middle of your tongue,
  especially in the morning?   ☑   ☐

D. BRAIN SYMPTOMS

Are the following symptoms present?
- Difficulties in concentration   ☑   ☐
- Decreased attention span   ☑   ☐
- Decreased memory   ☑   ☐
- Fogginess in the brain   ☑   ☐
- Drowsiness   ☑   ☐
- Incoordination   ☐   ☐
- Headaches   ☐   ☐
- Severe mood swings   ☐   ☐
- Depression   ☐   ☐
- Suicidal thoughts   ☐   ☐
- Anger and irritability   ☐   ☐

- Frustration ☐ ☐
- Being over defensive ☐ ☐

E. HORMONAL SYMPTOMS

Are the following symptoms present?
- PMS ☐ ☐
- Flare-up of yeast infections the week before the cycle ☐ ☐
- Loss of sexual desire ☐ ☐
- Impotence ☐ ☐
- Endometriosis ☐ ☐
- Menstrual irregularities ☐ ☐
- Flare-up of yeast infections after sexual intercourse ☐ ☐

F. OTHER SYMPTOMS

- Tightness in the chest ☐ ☐
- Palpitations ☐ ☐
- Urgency, frequency and burning on urination ☐ ☐
- Postnasal drip ☐ ☐
- Muscle pains, especially in the neck ☐ ☐
- Joint pains ☐ ☐
- Feeling hot inside and cold outside ☐ ☐
- Cold hands and feet ☐ ☐
- Water retention ☐ ☐
- Your doctor has told you it is all 'in your head' ☐ ☐
- Your doctor has told you it is 'psychosomatic' ☐ ☐
- Social isolation because of 'allergies' to food, smoke, fumes, allied to disbelief of your friends ☐ ☐
- Prostatitis ☐ ☐
- Difficulties swallowing ☐ ☐
- Sore throat ☐ ☐
- Burning of the eyelids ☐ ☐
- Itchy scaling skin lesions ☐ ☐

Note: all of these symptoms can be present in a thousand diseases. However, it is the simultaneous presence of a majority of them that is so specific for the Candida Syndrome.

Chapter 2
Diet Therapy

TREATING THE ENVIRONMENT

The first and best treatment of any disease is the prevention of it. We have to pay close attention to all the triggering factors. One that can be found in almost every patient is the over–use of antibiotics. We know that antibiotics are almost always prescribed for any infection, viral or bacterial. Doctors and patients have become so adjusted to the use of them, that they are almost prescribed or asked for as a reflex. Often it takes all my eloquence to convince a patient that not only should he not take an antibiotic for viral infections, but that it is hazardous to his health! In almost all the medical histories of my patients, I notice the over–use of antibiotics. One of my very first questions is "When did you last feel good and what happened?"; antibiotic intake is frequently the triggering factor. As we know, it is not the only factor. A doctor who accompanied his wife to my office questioned me about this. He said: "Antibiotics have been in use for 40 years and only now are we seeing this syndrome". Well first of all we probably never recognised the problem before (or even now), but what have we done to our environment, with continuous spraying of crop chemicals, car exhaust fumes, atomic plants; what have we done to our foods, with preservatives, low dosage antibiotics and hormones – to say nothing of stress levels in this decade of zombied yuppies, totally sold to the evils of the corporate environment!

Of course, there are sometimes indications for antibiotic intake. How do we then protect ourselves? By taking from the start, a high dose of Acidophilus (6 tbsp liquid as directed or a 1/4 tsp powder four times over the day). It is a pity that most doctors wait for the appearance of diarrhoea before suggesting Acidophilus, mostly in the form of yoghurt, which has a negligible concentration considering the purpose involved. Patients who are at that time on any anti-fungal medication should increase their dosage for the length of the antibiotic intake. Even for those patients who have not taken any medication, a low dosage of an anti-fungal medication intake is advised (page 82). Cortisone, the contraceptive pill, and immuno-suppressive medications should be avoided if at all possible. Hypothyroidism, diabetes mellitus and anaemia should be tested for and, if positive, corrected.

Yeast-containing foods have to be avoided totally at the beginning of any diet therapy. I remember a patient in my practice who used to perspire heavily and had a very low degree of energy. In fact, as he left my treatment table, his body would stick to the paper, he was perspiring so much. A mere seven-day anti-yeast diet completely changed this picture. Diet is discussed thoroughly later in the chapter.

It is also obvious that most patients of this type have to change their life styles. We have to realise that the changes have to come from within ourselves; a doctor is only there to give some guidelines. It is a bad start to declare as one of my patients did: "I give you one year to change me". I personally will not change anybody. Nobody can rescue you if there is not the determination and perseverance to want a healthier life. Because that is what your reward is. And do not believe those who say: "If I have to live this way, I would rather live a shorter life." Our survival instinct is our strongest instinct. What those people actually hope is that they can get away with abusing their bodies. Do not fall into this trap of denial! Five thousand years ago the Chinese already knew that worry and obsession about the past will injure the spleen and decrease its energy. People with Candidiasis unfortunately, or should I say logically, almost always fall into this category. They are mostly intelligent, very analytical and have an obsessive, compulsive nature. Because of the rejection that they all encounter, worry and frustration are constant growing feelings, starting the vicious cycle of spleen depression: the more they worry, the less energy is in the spleen, and the less energy, the more they will worry! And, that's where support groups can do a marvelous job. Finding people who have gone through the same suffering will convince Candida patients that one, they are not crazy and two, there is hope for recovery. Almost all patients are in a different stage of the disease and can give advice on how they manage their darkest moments. In the same way that the Alcoholics Anonymous movement is more successful in supporting alcoholics and curing alcoholism than any hospital treatment, support groups must, in the future, be a cornerstone in overcoming this terrible disease. While going through any change of life style, this provides a good opportunity to initiate psychotherapy and resolve all the issues left over from childhood. A good counsellor will help deal with frustration, depression, mood swings, suicidal thoughts and, above all, give you the attention you deserve, without judgement. Denial, misplacement and anger are frequently found in Candida patients. I remember a patient who was overweight and full of the Candida yeast; she could not bring herself to eat more healthily. She bought all the wrong foods for the rest of the family and, "because she could not let the food spoil", she participated (probably gladly) in this diet. Who was she fooling here?

As we have mentioned before, another Candida triggering factor is humidity and the presence of moulds. Both will decrease the energy in the spleen. How do we protect ourselves? Start by eliminating dampness in your home by checking the walls and roof for leaks. Waterproof walls and ceilings before painting. Paint instead of wallpapering to avoid the growth of moulds. Avoid carpets as floor covering but replace them with wood floors, vinyl or ceramic tile. Moulds grow in carpet, while the dust is also trapped, causing allergic reactions. Allow good air circulation in wardrobes by leaving space between hanging clothes. Check especially leather clothing, belts, shoes and luggage since moulds have a tendency to grow on these items. Keep bathrooms and laundry rooms well aired: spread out towels and washcloths for fast drying. In fact, in humid conditions, use air conditioning or a dehumidifier: moulds hate dry environments. And of course, avoid foods which contain moulds or are related to moulds such as mushrooms.

Sometimes the problem caused by presence of moulds can be so bad that there is nothing left to do but move. I know of a family that house moved to three different areas before they settled down in an 'ecological' house, free of carpets and gas stove, away from traffic and surrounded by woods. In the process, the husband lost his job and the whole family was isolated. Not everybody wants to make this sacrifice. It is easier when you live in a rented house, but what do you do when you live in an expensive house along a damp beach and your partner is healthy. There will be a lot of anger, frustration and despair for such patients because they are trapped in a predicament: it is too expensive to move, their partner does not want to move, and each time the patient enters the house, the symptoms are aggravated after an hour. These are not isolated cases, and they are hard to resolve!

The problem of being sensitive to the environment, for many patients, goes beyond the mould sensitivity. A great many women have become chemically sensitive to the fumes from gas stoves. In fact, gas is a major culprit, and I would advise anyone, especially Candida patients, to remove the gas pipes and replace the cooker with an electric one.

It is also a good idea to avoid airborne chemicals in the home such as waxes, mothballs, glue or anything else that evaporates. Avoid paint and varnish removers because of the presence of benzene, long time exposure to which is linked to leukaemia. Severe setbacks in Candida patients can be seen after exposure to freshly painted rooms. It is best to avoid sleeping in such rooms and move if you can to a friend's house for at least a couple of days. In fact it is best to paint in the spring, so that the windows can then be left open during summer. Candida patients will be able to detect paint fumes for three months after application.

Where are some of the favourite places for mould to grow? Basement, kitchen and bathroom harbour moulds in great quantities. Be sure to throw out those piles of old newspapers, magazines, clothes and leftovers, carpets and pillows. A favourite place in the bathroom is between shower or sink tiles and any less than water tight surround and these should be checked. In the kitchen be sure to check the surplus water tray on self-defrosting refrigerators. The growth of moulds is enhanced during the warm, humid summer months when the moulds mature and their spores are spread throughout the house.

Borax, a natural anti-mould agent, can be sprinkled in places of mould growth and is an efficient mould growth retardant. Another efficient anti-mould product is formaldehyde (37% solution), available from any pharmacy. Put one inch of formaldehyde solution in a container and use one container per 12 square feet of floor space. Candida patients should leave their homes for 48 hours while the formaldehyde is working. Upon their return, they should air the house out thoroughly.

Unfortunately, I have in my practice some patients who do not just have a problem with Candida, they seem to be allergic to 20th century life. All they can do is pack up and move into the desert to avoid pollution, synthetic materials and the like. But I believe there is another way; namely, to follow a strict way of life for a period of about a month. It is outlined below.

SPECIAL ONE-MONTH DIET

Rise at your regular time and drink at least two glasses of water with the juice of one lemon (the ideal detoxifier!). Take at this moment, 8-12 tablets of wheatgrass, 1-2 teaspoons juice of garlic BP and 1-2 teaspoons megadophilus.

Spend at least one hour taking a brisk walk, biking, jogging or any other outdoor activity. Practice breathing deeply. Be sure to start out slowly, each day increasing your pace. Shower with warm water, finish with cold.

At your usual breakfast time, mix 2 tablespoons of psyllium seeds (obtainable from a herbalist), with 4 oz of water or pineapple juice or papaya juice. Wash a bunch of parsley, mix it in your blender with just enough unsweetened pineapple juice to break it down to a nice thick drink. In cases of stomach irritation or hyperacidity, drink fresh cabbage juice (8 oz) before each meal.

For seven days your diet should consist only of beans (haricot, kidney, lentils) and green vegetables (lettuce, celery, avocado, peas, spinach, diced young turnips cooked with turnip greens, kale, collard). Greens cooked with chopped onions and garlic make a tasty side dish. Steam all your salads and vegetables; they are better tolerated this way.

Beans should be washed then place in a pan with enough water to cover and bring to the boil for 10 minutes. Drain, add fresh water and bring to a boil again, repeating this process three times. Place long cooking beans (brown, haricot or red kidney beans) in a slow cooker after boiling and cook on high for 12 HOURS, using one large onion, one bulb garlic, a little sea salt and cayenne.

Vary the bean diet toward the fifth day by adding fresh tomatoes and watch for any reaction. You can also eat rice crackers spread with a little mashed avocado during the first week.

Take your juice of garlic and acidophilus after each meal. If you wish to have three meals, your meal times should be 6 am, 1 pm and 5.30 pm. The ideal is two meals a day with nothing after 3 pm. Only fruit and grains are allowed in the evening, mainly fresh pineapple, avocado, apricots and papaya or juices, if they do not contain artificial sweeteners.

The most important facet in this 'cave man' diet is plenty of water! By the early morning to the time you retire at night, you should have drunk 6 pints of water. Do not drink water with your meals, or 20 minutes before or 1 hour after meals.

Candida sufferers all need some help with digestion: Bromelain, an enzyme extracted from pineapple, 2 tablets with each meal, is an excellent help. Other supplements for these patients are L-Tryptophan, a valuable sleep aid, taken 1 hour before going to bed adding a complex carbohydrate food such as banana. Together with another amino acid, Thyrosin, taken as directed, it is the ideal way to fight depression and mood swings.

Goat's milk is very valuable for high quality absorption. It has been found especially valuable for those suffering from aller-gies. It has a calming effect on the most nervous individual. A 4 oz portion before you exercise helps keep down the garlic, 4 oz at meals with 8 oz before retiring benefits those losing weight.

Fruits, vegetables, nuts and grains make the ideal diet. From too much sugar in our usual 'junk' diet, our body at first has a hard time handling the natural sugars in high sugar fruits. For this reason, pineapple, grapefruit, lemon and avocado seem to be the only ones tolerated in the first week. Other fruits should be added very slowly; peel your fruit unless it is grown organi-cally. Start adding grain the second week to avoid allergic reactions. Do not eat sweet vegetables such as corn and potatoes together, at least not at the start. All meat and animal products are hard to digest, contain no fibre and are unnecessary at this moment in your diet.

It is extremely important to use up to 8 tablespoons of juice of garlic; gradually, you will be able to cut down to 6 and 4 tablespoons. A good combination is 6 tablespoons juice of garlic with 6 garlic capsules.

As you can see, this diet is not easy, but life for Candida patients is never easy. They are allergic to practically every food, supplement, cigarette smoke, household cleansers and house plants (because the soil plants are grown in encourages the growth of moulds). Going into shops is impossible, they can only wear 100% cotton clothes, and perfumes can cause serious reactions. Car exhaust fumes can induce asthma attacks and swollen throats.

It is frightening that the food we eat, the water we drink, medicine we take, clothing we wear, as well as the air we breath at home, work or school, constitute not only our environment, but in many cases become a real menace to our physical and mental well being. What can we do to stay healthy in a chemical world?

Good health is not a gift, it is something we must help search for and find. As chronic illness overtakes us, basic rules become more and more important: eat organically, read the labels, eat less sugar and salt, and bring a variety of fruit and vegetables to our diet.

Sixty per cent of the leading causes of death are linked to our over-consumption of fats, cholesterol, sugar, salt and alcohol. Cutting off the fat on our meat will allow us to avoid most of the chemicals. As mentioned before, chickens are fed antibiotics, cattle and pigs are given hormones. These powerful chemicals end up in our bodies in such high levels that they can be measured in laboratories. Be aware of fish as a meat substitute since preservatives are often added at sea to keep fish fresh until it can be brought to the processor. Fish caught in colder climates where this is not needed are safer. The best fish to buy in this respect are probably salmon, halibut and cod, all caught in cold waters.

Remember also that 'natural' is not organic. Only food grown without commercial sprays and fertilizers should be labelled organic. Unless food is labelled organic, you should not be paying more for it. Statements such as 'no chemicals or preservatives added' on labels often refer to food that has been commercially grown.

Call your local Water Authority and ask what additives are in the local supply. These additives are often a source of sensitivity. Use water bottled in glass, not plastic. If the best you can drink is bottled in plastic, pour it into a sterile glass jar and leave the top off for a short while so that any chemicals from the plastic can escape.

Some other handy advice in your kitchen:

Use stainless steel, iron, glass or ceramic cookware rather than non-stick pans.

Cook beans in a slow cooker after boiling for 10 minutes.

Rotate foods by spacing each one five days apart. By spacing these foods, you are actually performing the most simple allergy test. You eliminate a certain food (wheat, milk, corn or beef, for example) for four days; eat it on the fifth day and observe any adverse reactions. Under these specific conditions, adverse reactions are noted within minutes.

Cooking sometimes makes food more tolerable for the highly sensitive. You can freeze leftovers and eat them in rotation five days later.

Try fasting for 24 hours. If this is difficult, it is almost certain that you have some food allergy.

As the illness grows, you may become addicted to smoking, alcohol and drugs. Food you become allergic to can do the same things. They too can fool you into thinking you need them.

Sugar is the best example. After consuming it, for an hour or two you might feel better (relieving the apparent hypoglycaemia), even though it is the source of your problem. When you remove an important food that acts as an adverse reactor, you will experience withdrawal symptoms. But feel good about it, you have 'unmasked' the enemy because removing it from your diet will make a big difference to how you feel.

It is wise to avoid those who smoke or wear hairspray or perfumes. Wash your clothes without detergents but use mild soap, borax and soda instead. Wash windows with vinegar water.

Above all, develop a sense of humour and guard against self-pity! Learn to listen to your body because environmental illness will affect each individual in its own way.

There is another important factor for 'super-allergic' people: positive ions. Ions are submicroscopic particles that have no taste and do not stimulate our sense organs in any way. Positive ions are produced by heating air, by air moving past an obstruction such as a bend in an air conditioning duct and by synthetic fabrics; they are easily found in crowds of people. Do you recognize this situation? This is exactly what we find in most of our modern buildings, from workplaces to homes.

Negative ions on the other hand, seem to be the most beneficial ions since they carry an extra electron which makes them negative. Where do we find these ions? Falling water is a natural source of negative ions and we all remember the good feelings associated with showers, or being in the neighbourhood of the ocean or waterfalls. Unfortunately, the positive ions have a strong hold in nature too; they are associated with the 'named' winds around the world: 'Santa Ana' in Southern California, the 'Foehn' in Europe and the 'Sharav' in Israel. At least 30% of the world population are thought to be suffering from these weather–related conditions.

It has been found that humans produce a hormone-like substance called serotonin under the stress of too many positive ions. What does serotonin do? It is a neuro-transmitter, involved in the induction of sleep. However, there can be disastrous consequences when too much serotonin is formed: we will seem sleepy and without energy all the time. Extreme fatigue, depression, irritability and decreased breathing capacity are present in all such patients as well as in hyperactive people who swing to deep depressions. This situation becomes a little more understandable when we know that the general charge on earth is negative, while the charge in the atmosphere is positive. This positive ion layer is moved tidally by the gravitational effect of the moon and the result is an increase in positive ions, with disastrous consequences for weather-sensitive people.

So should we breathe only negative ions? In general, they have no side-effects, but in people with depressed levels of serotonin, they can lead to insomnia and hyper-alertness. This hyper-alert stage does not allow any cell repair and disturbs the natural organ clock. But being exposed to an air ionizer, even for the whole day, will not have that negative effect. Quite the contrary, you will have added protection against viruses and bacteria since they will be pulled out of the air like other dust particles by the negative ions.

Once we have taken care of the triggering factors, we can start our battle against Candidiasis. And, it is a major battle requiring all the troops we have available. Seven major steps will win this fight: 1) STARVE THE CANDIDA; 2) KILL THE CANDIDA; 3) EVACUATE THE DEAD CANDIDA OR TOXINS; 4) AVOID SPREADING TO THE BLOOD STREAM (SYSTEMIC CANDIDIASIS); 5) REPLACE THE NORMAL FLORA; 6) BOOST THE IMMUNE SYSTEM; 7) REPLACE THE MISSING SUPPLEMENTS. Step by step, we will discuss each of these weapons against yeast. It has amazed me time and time again that people do perhaps three steps well but pay no attention to the others. Inevitably, they will fail to cure the disease, arrive at a plateau in their healing or delay the recovery from this debilitating disease.

THE ANTI-YEAST DIET

The first line of defence against Candida is diet. Diet has always and should always be the starting point of a healthy life. In ancient China there were different classes of doctors. The highest in esteem was the nutritional doctor since he prevented disease from appearing. The one lowest in esteem was the doctor who took care of the patient once the disease had already appeared. This is exactly what the majority of the present doctors do. And it does not look as if any improvement is in sight: insurance companies do not pay for inexpensive preventive medicine, but see no problem with reimbursing large bills for private hospital treatment. I have read an interview with a Nobel prize winner in medicine who claimed that the importance of food is highly exaggerated and plays a minimal role in maintaining our health. I am sorry to say so, but my grandmother had more common sense. Food is still the fuel that your motor runs on, and if I have the choice, I prefer to go for quality!

Diet is very important, and at the same time, very difficult and frustrating. However, if a patient feels that they do not make any progress or come to a plateau during the treatment, the first reflex is to take a closer look at the food intake. Many times a patient thinks they are eating all the right things, but upon closer examination, many foods can be found to cause yeast growth. Therefore, the patient does not make any break-through and returns to their previous bad eating habits, since "this boring diet does not make any difference". And they promptly reward themselves with ice cream and cake: the rest is history, and Candida wins the game!

Each time I start explaining the content of this diet, I will invariably hear: "I may as well starve, there is nothing more left to eat". Maybe so at first sight. What it really requires for most people is a total change from their convenient junk food diet to one that requires more imagination and work. And forget par-ties and eating out. That's why this disease is such an isolating disease; the patient actually transmits the disease to the partner. The partner becomes a prisoner of the house, since the Candida patient cannot go out, cannot go to cinemas or parties because of environmental factors. Of course, this is not always taken well! And the poor Candida patient receives more rejection, anger and impatience. The vicious circle is then closed and many of these patients have an enormous amount of anger and frustra-tion, something they can best deal with in a support group, led by a competent psychologist.

Basically, the diet itself is low in carbohydrates and high in protein. Before going into detail, some important facts have to be pointed out. First, avoid raw and cold foods! Climatic damp-ness spells doom for the spleen; cold raw foods cause a form of interior dampness. The moment we are aware of 'damp' we know it means trouble for the spleen. I have seen patients who could not lose weight despite being on what they thought was a healthy diet. They were eating only salads and raw vegetables and could not lose one pound; some even gained weight. So limit salads and avoid raw vegetables for the time being.

Secondly, do not eat leftovers. When food is stored in the refrigerator, moulds have a great opportunity to grow over-night! Freeze your leftovers and reheat them.

Thirdly, rotate your foods. The easiest way to acquire aller-gies to food is to continually eat the same things. Examples of rotation diets are outlined later in the chapter.

Furthermore, if you start this diet, do it a hundred per cent!

Doing it halfway will only give you headaches, frustration and anger. You will not make any progress, your yeast cells will keep on growing; so will your cravings and any other symptoms.

As we have already mentioned, the increased growth of yeast before the menstrual cycle is due to progesterone levels and yeast intake has to be extremely well watched around this period. Try to exercise, treat yourself to something pleasant (a walk in the country, a film if you can, or a phone call to a good friend who can give you some support).

And last but not least, remember that this is not a diet that will go on for the rest of your life. Do not think you will never again be able to touch cheese, dairy products or breads. The better start you give yourself, the shorter the diet period will be. Usually, I say to the patient: "Try it very strictly for seven days". Everybody can do it for that period and usually it will be enough for a major change in the patient's symptoms. Once they feel the benefit of this diet change, they are positively stimulated to go on with it. As the patient gets better, blood 'allergies' will disppear, they will be able to add new foods week by week, and gradually break away from monotonous diet.

The quickest way to recovery is to follow this diet as strictly as possible for one month. After this period, certain foods will be re-introduced one by one: this way, we will recognise an 'allergic' reaction right away. The body will often react to that particular food within half an hour. Mostly, you will experience headaches, bloating and sudden fatigue. The same happens when patients are 'cheating' on their diet. Some of the foods that can be tried first will be some cereals, some more fruits and oatmeals. But please stay away for a longer time from wines, champagne, dairy products and, of course, SUGAR. Do you want to visualise what happens in your gastro–intestinal system when you add sugar? When you bake bread and dissolve yeast in hot water, nothing happens. The moment you add sugar to this mixture, it starts growing and bubbling, the smell is more activated and it warms up. Can you imagine all this happening in your poor bowels? No wonder bloating and gas are an immediate reaction. On the other hand, cheating once on your diet does not automatically put you back where you started from. You will merely go through a short period of die-off, a sign of the continuous battle between the yeast and your body's defenders.

Do not forget, however, that at some point in your diet you will crave the very foods that created the condition. If you understand that you desire the very thing that is being eliminated, you can better overcome this pressing craving. Be clear in your commitment to healing and take an honest look at the 'benefits' you may be getting from being sick.

Forbidden foods (yeast foods)

Breads are almost always craved by Candida patients and should be excluded from the diet. This includes wheat, as well as rye breads, even if yeast-free. Other main culprits are: dairy products, cheese of all kinds, cottage cheese, mushrooms (a fungus!), wine and champagne. Other yeast-containing foods are: apple, pear, grapes, vinegar–based condiments (except pepper, paprika, onion and garlic), salad dressing (except oil and lemon), tomato sauce, barbecue sauce, teas (including herbal teas), coffee (including decaffeinated), whisky, cognac, oatmeals, cereals, horseradish, biscuits, cakes, honey, sugar, artificial sweeteners, fruit juices, ice cream, almost any fruit (except some tropical ones), dried fruits.

Some of the above nutrients do not contain yeasts but they will enhance the growth of the yeast cells.

High carbohydrate foods are also to be limited: lima beans, potatoes, winter squash, lentils, popcorn, pumpkin, peas and barley.

Allowed foods

We start off with plain water: sometimes it is very advantageous to add lemon juice (five drops in a glass of water) in order to free the body from any dead toxins.

Only two teas are allowed: Taheebo tea (also known as Pau D'Arco tea), a Brazilian herbal tea. This tea is known to have natural anti-fungal properties. Two to three cups daily (not more in order to avoid too heavy a die-off) will often clear the head. To improve its taste, lemon or cinnamon can be added. Another important tea is black walnut leaf tea (obtainable from herbalists), known for its eliminating effects on the worms and parasites frequently seen in Candida patients.

In cases of constipation, papaya juice mixed half and half with water can be allowed.

Special attention should be paid to cranberry juice, sometimes referred to as 'nature's healing cocktail'. Cystitis-like symptoms are a frequent symptom with Candida patients. For more than fifty years, cranberry products have been used in our diets to control the growth of bacteria in the urine and also to reduce strong odour in urine. Cranberry is a native American product that is used traditionally to make sauces and drinks. The fruit is very acidic so that its juice is not easily taken raw and to improve the taste, it is customarily diluted with water. Cranberry juice concentrate is available in health food shops. Natural cranberries diluted with water do not contain added sugar or sweeteners. Another form, also available in health food shops, is cranberry juice concentrate in soft gelatine capsules. Cranberries are a source of vitamins A, C, B-complex and several minerals such as potassium, manganese, iron and calcium. It is also a strong inhibitor of bacterial adherence preventing foreign invading bacteria from attaching to the urinary tract lining.

Corn, popcorn, rice (for preference, brown rice and wild rice), eggs, rice cakes, buckwheat, millet, gooseberries, fresh meats (except beef and pork), all seafood, all vegetables (steamed or stir-fried), all nuts, unsalted, raw (except peanuts and pistachios), all seeds, salads with oil and lemon dressing, yams, beans, butter, nut butters (except peanut), rice bran, condiments (see rotation diet, page 43) rice noodles, Japanese buckwheat noodles, goat's milk, tropical fruits (pineapple, papaya, mango, kiwi, banana, honeydew melon, but no cantaloupe or watermelon, guava or lemons), wheatgrass juice, or wheatgrass tablets and powder (an organic product, extremely high in chlorophyll, beta–carotene, minerals and an excellent source of dietary fibre), corn tortillas, corn chips, goat cheese.

KEY FOODS PROFILE

BREWER'S YEAST

Unfortunately, brewer's yeast seems to have become a victim of Candida fear. I say unfortunately because, by omitting brewer's yeast from our supplements, we cut out a wonderful natural supplement which is an aid to our immune system. And we know that boosting the immune system is the ultimate goal of our therapy. Research studies have shown that relapses in Candida patients occur because of failure to strengthen the immune system. So let's have a closer look at brewer's yeast before we decide to ban it out of our lives.

Brewer's yeast is one of the best sources of the entire vitamin B family. Even more important, it provides us with chromium or Glucose Tolerance Factor; without it, the body cannot make use of its major fuel, blood sugar. Good news for Candida patients is that brewer's yeast is also a superb source of protein, being rich in amino acids. There is even help for memory loss and concentration difficulties experienced by Candida patients; lecithin, a natural source of choline, is abundantly present. The antioxidant, selenium, and other nutritional factors are provided for use by the body.

Boosting the immune system to keep the yeast cells away is the first line of defence in beating Candida. That system needs nutritional ammunition and brewer's yeast that can do more for our body's defence mechanism than any other natural food!

POPCORN

What's fun to make, low in calories, does not harm the teeth, is economical and good for you? Popcorn, an all-American discovery. It is a type of corn with small hard kernels. The plants have the same food value as other varieties of corn. Each kernel contains about 30% moisture which will change to steam when heated to 400°F (200°C). A cup sized portion of buttered popcorn has about 40 calories. It is part of a balanced diet and not a junk food at all. Even with a little added butter, it has only 65 calories compared to 200 calories for four chocolate chip cookies. According to the American Dental Association, popcorn does not contribute to dental caries. It is a safe and nutritious snack. In fact, it may help teeth and gums because of its cleansing and massaging effect. It is also high in fibre; adding bulk to the diet thus preventing constipation and some chronic diseases of the large intestine, and decreasing the appetite by causing a full-up feeling. Fibre in the diet is also believed to protect against colon cancer.

BEANS

Everyone seems interested in the nutritional value of beans these days. They are an excellent source of protein and have a longer shelf-life than most animal, vegetable and fruit products. They contain no cholesterol and 80% less total fat than lean beef. They are an excellent source of minerals. Cooking beans is a little complex since they do require long cooking times. One way to decrease the cooking time is to presoak the beans overnight; alternatively, plunge them into boiling water for two minutes and then soak them for one hour. After this, beans need to be boiled for a minimum of 10 minutes and simmered for two hours to make them tender enough to eat. Beans are an excellent low-fat source of protein and combined with rice or corn they serve as the primary protein source for much of the world's population. One of the problems with eating beans is that they cause distension in many individuals. This is due to the non-digestible carbohydrates in the beans which are fermented by bacteria and yeasts. If you like beans, but have problems with intestinal gas (which most Candida patients have), activated charcoal can help. Twenty to fifty grams taken orally can greatly relieve the problem.

Other gas producing foods which respond to the same remedy are apples, bananas, Brussels sprouts, broccoli, cauliflower, celery, milk products, onions, raisins, prunes and wheat germ.

RICE

Rice is truly one of the world's great treasures. For more than half the earth's population, rice is the staff of life. Asia produces more than 90% of the world's rice. Newly harvested rice is covered by an unedible husk which is removed from the dried grains by pounding and shaking. What remains is brown rice. If the kernels are then rubbed mechanically until the bran is removed, we have white polished rice. The bran coating on brown rice contains many nutrients, which can be critical where rice is a major source of calories. Rice is also the least allergenic of all grains. Wheat triggers four times as many allergic reactions, corn three times as many. Washing or soaking rice removes valuable B vitamins.

AMARANTH (*Amaranthus hybridus* and other varieties)

Amaranth, a little-known crop of the Americas, is grown either as a grain crop or as a leafy vegetable. Despite its obscurity, it offers important promise for feeding the world's hungry. This broad-leafed plant is one of the few non-grasses that produce significant amounts of edible 'cereal' grain. It grows vigorously, resisting drought, heat and pests. It is also a beautiful crop with brilliantly coloured leaves, stems and flowers. The seed heads occur in massive numbers, sometimes more than 50,000 to a plant. Amaranth has two big advantages: it has a very high protein content, 16%, compared to the 12% of wheat, 7-10% of rice and 9% of maize. The seed contains protein of unusual quality, high in the amino acid lysine. It is therefore a nutritional complement to conventional cereals. When heated, the tiny amaranth grains pop and can be eaten as a snack; they taste like a nut-flavoured popcorn. Amaranth is high in the amino acids lysine and tryptophan; corn is high in leucine so when amaranth flour is mixed with corn flour, the two form a perfectly balanced combination because the essential amino acids that are deficient in one are abundant in the other.

GOOSEBERRIES

Calcium deficiency, a condition that often manifests itself by osteoporosis of the bones and poor mineralization of the teeth has an excellent natural remedy, gooseberries. A 100 gram (3.5 oz) portion of gooseberries contains 564 mg of calcium, an extraordinary amount considering that the same amount of apples contains 8 mg, dates 52 mg and cow's milk 116 to 175 mg.

At first glance, it would seem that most people, given their relatively high consumption of milk and other dairy products, would easily get all the calcium their systems need from their daily fare. But alas, this is not so.

Only about 10% of elements in the cow's milk purchased at your supermarket can be readily assimilated. Of course, for a Candida patient, the problem becomes even more acute: dairy products are among the forbidden foods, hence the vogue for calcium pills which are selling so well at health food stores. The usual dose is one gram of calcium per day, of which at most 100 mg will be absorbed by the body. Compare that with 200 grams of gooseberries where the amount of calcium absorbed will be 1.28 grams.

The plant was introduced to Western Europe by Anne of Russia. Gooseberries were her beauty and health secret. A French clinician who has studied and used food plants for many ailments that do not respond to drugs, has written that gooseberries are a good appetiser, good for the digestion, a natural laxative in sufficient quantities, and a diuretic.

QUINOA (Chenopodium quinoa)

This is one of the 'rediscovered' foods and quite similar in properties to amaranth. It is a grain that comes from the Andean Mountain region of South America. Its origin is ancient: it was one of the three staple foods (along with corn and potatoes) of the Inca civilization. It is referred to, respectfully, as the Mother Grain.

Quinoa contains more protein than any other grain: an average of 16%. It is, in fact, a complete protein food, with an essential amino acid balance close to the ideal. It is high in lysine, methionine and cystine, thus boosting the food value of other grains when combined with them. Although no single food can supply all the life-sustaining nutrients, quinoa comes closer than any other food.

And, if this is not enough, listen to the following advantages. It is light, tasty and easy to digest. Its flour is low in gluten and it can be used for most baked goods. It is easy and quick to prepare: a whole dish takes just 15 minutes to prepare. It is perfect in the summertime: quinoa's lightness, combined with its versatility in cold dishes like salads and desserts, make it an ideal source of good warm weather nutrition. Cooked quinoa grain expands almost five times compared to about three times for brown rice. It is an excellent source of nutrition for children and nursing mothers.

Nuts and Seeds

There is growing evidence that seeds and nuts were the major staples of early humans. Archaeological excavations show that pre-historic men and women frequently used the seeds and nuts of a wide variety of wild plants, especially in the northern climates. The season during which food could be gathered was short, and as seeds and nuts are easily storable, they were no doubt a stable and convenient food source. As agriculture began, cereal grains, the cultivated seeds of grasses, have gradually replaced nuts in importance. However, nutritious nuts are used as 'famine foods' by many cultures and, even today, many primitive people depend upon seeds and nuts for a large part of their nourishment. For the Candida patient, nuts provide an excellent snack, as long as they are eaten unsalted and raw, or at least not honey roasted. What nuts and seeds are available?

Let's start with the nuts to avoid: peanuts and pistachios. The peanut is not a nut, rather it is a legume or bean. Peanuts are mainly grown for their oil, except in the USA where 50% of the crop goes into peanut butter. Peanuts are susceptible to the aflatoxin mould, one of the most powerful toxins known. Roasting does not destroy the mould so natural foods manufacturers retest the nuts before using them in peanut butter. Because of its mould content, peanuts are forbidden for the Candida patient.

Pistachios are the seeds of an evergreen which has been grown in the Mediterranean region for over 5000 years. The seeds can be dyed for eye appeal, although natural food shops usually stock only the undyed ones. Since they are almost always salted and roasted, this excludes them from the yeast diet.

Chestnuts are allowed in small quantities: they are low in calories, but also low in protein and high in starch or carbohydrates. They should be eaten fresh (boiled) but not dried as this makes them sweeter.

Pine-nuts come from the Mediterranean and China and contain more protein than any other nut. They are fairly high in price and have a definite piney taste. One of the most popular nuts on sale in natural food shops is the walnut. Their probable origin is Persia, although they have been under cultivation for so many centuries that their exact place of origin is unknown. Some walnuts are darker than others; the dark ones have grown on the side of the tree that received more sunshine. But outside colour is not as important as the colour inside which should be white and clean.

Hazelnuts are another delicious nut. They are often used as a symbol of love and are the most common nut tree in England and Spain. They have a pleasant taste, and can be eaten raw as a snack or used in cooking.

Almonds are the oldest and most widely grown of all nuts and are closely related to the peach. Their shells help protect the nut against oxidation and rancidity. Good almonds have a smooth and even shape with an intact skin. Almonds become more digestible after roasting; if raw they should be eaten in small quantities.

Cashews are the fruit of a tropical evergreen, originally from Brazil. Traditionally, the fruits were picked by hand and the nuts removed and dried in the sun, then placed among burning logs where the heat would crack them open. Their 45% fat content makes them difficult to store for any length of time, and the raw nut tends to be indigestible. Dry-roasted cashews, however, are becoming increasingly popular.

Seeds are another delicious snack for Candida patients: sesame seeds, sunflower seeds and pumpkin seeds are all suitable. Sesame is the oldest known herb grown for its seeds. They are extremely nutritious and highly versatile.

Nutritionally, sesame seeds are real power houses. They contain over 35% protein and have twice as much calcium as milk. Since dairy products are out for Candida patients, these seeds are therefore a welcome source of much needed calcium. Most of the seeds sold in natural food shops come from Central America.

Sunflower seeds were once used extensively by American Indians who made seed bread and drinks. They are nutritionally similar to sesame seeds but are even higher in protein and phosphorus, although they have less calcium. Flourine, vita-mins D, E and B-complex are other plus points. The important thing about these seeds is to check their condition: they should be firm, not too hard and with few broken seeds. Pumpkin seeds are also highly nutritious since they contain up to 30% protein.

MILLET

This is the ideal grain for the Candida patient. As stressed before, the root of the problem is a deficiency of energy in the Spleen-Pancreas. Millet is said to be good for the spleen and stomach (known as the Yin-Yang unit) and because of its alka-line nature, it is good for people who suffer from acidosis. It is considered to have the most complete protein of all the grains and is high in minerals. The variety most commonly sold in health food shops is pearl millet.

SWEETENERS

One thing that everyone agrees on is that white sugar should be removed from the diet. As soon as we decide to give up this 'poison', we begin searching for 'natural' alternatives that can satisfy our sweet tooth. Unfortunately, no such sweetener ex-ists. We should keep in mind that there is no evidence that the use of sweeteners is necessary to maintain health. On the other hand, sugar intake is linked to arthritis, hypertension, obesity, diabetes and dental caries. Unfortunately, today we consume over fifteen times the sugar we did 100 years ago.

All sweeteners are concentrated simple sugars and, as such, cannot be considered whole foods. Natural sweeteners have many of the same effects on the body as white sugar. Common sense tells us that if we eat whole foods, the vitamins, minerals and enzymes present will allow smooth metabolism of the sugars contained in them. The best way for the body to take in sugar is through the digestion of complex carbohydrates: the starch from grains, vegetables and fruits is digested slowly, releasing sugar into the blood gradually. This prevents the insulin overload and adrenal exhaustion that accompanies the ingestion of concentrated simple sugars. The Candida patient can get his sweet taste from tropical fruits such as pineapple, papaya, mango, banana, honeydew melon and kiwi. They are best eaten once a day, not combined with any other food: they make the ideal breakfast. Do not eat fruit all day, however, since the total amount of sugar intake will be too high. Do not eat dried fruits since the main sugar in dried pineapple, for instance, is sucrose: it may even amount to over 50% of the product. Another important aspect of tropical fruits is their digestive enzyme content: papain and bromelain are two powerful enzymes, found in papaya and pineapple. During the first month of the diet, molasses, honey, corn syrup, maple syrup and malt should be excluded from the diet. From all these sweeteners, maple syrup is the most organic and can be introduced into the diet after one month.

FOOD ROTATION, DAILY MENUS AND RECIPES

Food rotation

DAY ONE	DAY TWO	DAY THREE	DAY FOUR
Watercress	Brussels sprouts	Cabbage	Chives
Artichoke	Endive	Iceberg lettuce	Green pepper
Parsley	Lettuce	Spinach	Beetroot
Asparagus	Broccoli	Celery	Potato
Leeks	Corn	Alfalfa sprouts	Sweet potato
Avocado	Courgette	Cucumber	Egg white
Yellow squash	Aubergine	Pumpkin	Calves' liver
Carrots	Onions	Turnips	Anchovy
Tomatoes	Chicken	Duck	Lobster
Radish	Turkey	Lamb	Salmon
Beef	Cod	Veal	Shrimp
Egg yolk	Halibut	Crab	Tuna
Pork	Scallops	Herring	Lima beans
Mackerel	Swordfish	Sea Bass	String beans
Sardines	Dried beans	Trout	Lemon
Sole	Millet	Soya beans	Nutmeg
Haricot beans	Brown rice	Wild rice	Black pepper
Lentils	Bay leaf	Kelp	Safflower
Basil	Dill	Unsalted butter	
Cayenne	Ginger	Mustard seeds	
Garlic	White pepper	Paprika	
Lime	Sesame	Poppy seeds	
Olive Oil		Thyme	
Pepper		Gooseberries	
Chilli			

Daily Menus

──────────────── 1 ────────────────

BREAKFAST	*2 ricecakes spread with cashew butter*
LUNCH	*Boiled or braised chicken with lemon and vegetables*
SNACK	*3 small packets of corn chips*
DINNER	*2 ricecakes spread with cashew butter*
SNACK	*Handful of raw cashews*

──────────────── 2 ────────────────

BREAKFAST	*½ mango and whole kiwi*
LUNCH	*Veal chop sautéed in butter* *Steamed ½ corn cob, beetroot, carrot, asparagus*
SNACK	*Large package of corn chips*
DINNER	*Scampi sautéed in butter and garlic* *Steamed green beans, marrow and two slices of yam*

──────────────── 3 ────────────────

BREAKFAST	*½ mango and ½ banana*
SNACK	*1 ricecake spread with cashew butter*
LUNCH	*2 large bowls homemade lentil soup (onion, carrot, Chinese leaves, chicken leg, garlic and lentils)* *Boiled artichoke*
DINNER	*Braised chicken leg and steamed vegetables*
SNACK	*Pumpkin seeds and raw cashews*
NOTE	*For drinks, water and tea (Pau D'Arco) only allowed*

BREAKFAST   *1 kiwi and 1½ bananas*

LUNCH   *Baked or grilled red mullet*
            Steamed vegetables

DINNER   *150 g/ 6 oz buckwheat*
            Steamed ½ cob corn, asparagus and ¼ marrow or
            acorn squash

SNACK   *Bowl of freshly made popcorn*

───────────── 5 ─────────────

BREAKFAST   *¼ honeydew melon*

LUNCH   *Small piece of sturgeon, sword fish or tuna*
            sautéed with lime, dill and pepper, steamed
            carrots and asparagus

SNACK   *2 ricecakes*

DINNER   *Tuna steak marinated with olive oil, dill and*
            garlic, baked potato with butter, salt and pepper
            and corn on the cob

SNACK   *3 ricecakes*

───────────── 6 ─────────────

BREAKFAST   *1 kiwi and ¼ honeydew melon*

LUNCH   *3 ricecakes, cold poached salmon, corn chips*

SNACK   *1 kiwi and ½ papaya*

DINNER   *½ chicken (lean only), braised with lemon*
            Brown and wild rice, steamed herbs and green
            beans

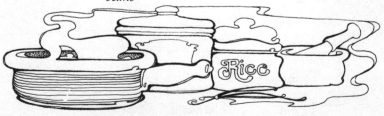

BREAKFAST	¼ honeydew melon 2 rice or wild rice cakes
LUNCH	½ braised chicken 1 small yam Lettuce salad
DINNER	2-egg spinach omelette 150 g/ 6 oz buckwheat
SNACK	2 ricecakes spread with butter

BREAKFAST	¼ honeydew melon and 75 g/3 oz bilberries
LUNCH	2-egg onion omelette, 120 g/4½ oz brown rice, raw spinach salad with oil and lemon
DINNER	Stir fried turkey, onion and broccoli with brown rice

BREAKFAST	2 soft boiled eggs and 150 g/6 oz buckwheat
SNACK	1 packet corn chips
LUNCH	Braised tuna marinated in oil, lemon, basil Steamed beet greens and marrow or crookneck squash
DINNER	Poached salmon Steamed mange tout and green beans
SNACK	2 ricecakes spread with almond butter

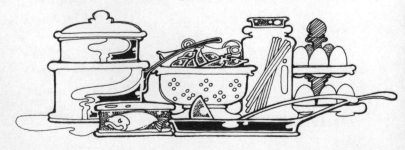

BREAKFAST	½ mango and 1 kiwi
SNACK	1 small packet corn chips
LUNCH	2 braised chicken thighs without skin and garlic Steamed beetroot, marrow and beet greens
DINNER	Salad of spinach and round-heart lettuce with 1 chopped hard boiled egg and ricecake croûtons. Dressing of garlic, lemon juice, olive oil, pepper
SNACK	Handful of dry roasted cashews

—— 11 ——

BREAKFAST	½ mango, ⅛ honeydew melon and 1 kiwi
LUNCH	Salmon steak, sautéed with butter, basil and garlic Steamed asparagus and mange tout
SNACK	1 small bag each potato crisps and corn chips
DINNER	Pan-fried cod or haddock with brown rice
SNACK	Buckwheat rice crackers

—— 12 ——

BREAKFAST	Rice cakes or brown rice cereal
LUNCH	Green salad with lemon Boiled potatoes and broccoli Grilled salmon
SNACK	2 ricecakes with roasted almond butter
DINNER	Baked red mullet Courgettes sautéed with onion, garlic, fresh coriander leaves and sunflower seeds in butter Brown rice
SNACK	1 ricecake with cashew butter

BREAKFAST	*1 halved papaya sprinkled with lime juice*
SNACK	*1 large packet of corn chips*
LUNCH	*Lentil soup*
DINNER	*½ braised chicken* *Steamed marrow, asparagus, beetroot*
SNACK	*Handful of raw cashews*

--- 14 ---

BREAKFAST	*2 ricecakes spread thin with cashew butter*
LUNCH	*Red mullet, sautéed with butter, garlic and basil* *Steamed beetroot, marrow, mange tout, leek*
DINNER	*Baked potato with butter and pepper, stir fried* *onion, asparagus and mange tout*
SNACK	*Buckwheat and brown rice crackers*

--- 15 ---

BREAKFAST	*Honeydew melon (⅛), ½ small mango and few* *raspberries*
LUNCH	*1 large packet corn chips*
DINNER	*½ braised chicken with lemon* *Cos lettuce and dressing* *Baked potato with butter*

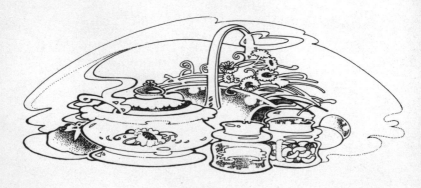

16

BREAKFAST — *Ricecakes or brown rice cereal*

LUNCH — *Small piece of sturgeon, sword fish or tuna sautéed in butter*
Corn on the cob and one beetroot, steamed

SNACK — *2 small packets corn chips*

DINNER — *Stir fried bok choy (Chinese cabbage) onion and broccoli and rice*

SNACK — *Handful of sunflower seeds and raw almonds*

BREAKFAST — *2-egg omelette*

LUNCH — *Cos salad with oil and lemon juice dressing*
½ braised chicken

DINNER — *2 packets health crackers and 1 packet (small) corn chips followed later by 1 ricecake spread thinly with cashew butter*

BREAKFAST — *Cooked brown rice cereal made with water*

SNACK — *Almonds, raw and unsalted*

LUNCH — *75 g/3 oz sturgeon, sword fish or tuna sautéed in butter and fresh dill with spinach salad - olive oil and lemon dressing*

DINNER — *1 rib steak on the bone (trimmed of fat)*
Baked potato and 2 baby aubergines sautéed in garlic, basil and olive oil

BREAKFAST *1 banana*

SNACK *Raw cashew nuts and sesame seeds*

LUNCH *Scallops, sautéed with pine-nuts and chives in butter*
Steamed mixed vegetables

BREAKFAST *½ papaya*

LUNCH *½ braised chicken, briefly marinated in lemon, ginger and olive oil*
Steamed beetroot, marrow or yellow squash

DINNER *Corn on the cob, 1 crookneck squash, 5 tiny carrots, steamed brown rice*

BREAKFAST *½ papaya and 1 banana*

LUNCH *Tuna sautéed in butter and raw spinach salad with garlic, olive oil and lemon juice*

SNACK *Small packet corn tortilla chips without salt*

DINNER *Pan-fried cod or haddock, buttered carrots and potatoes*

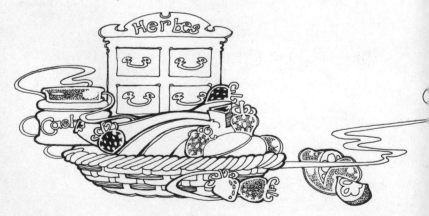

BREAKFAST	*¼ papaya and a handful of strawberries*
SNACK	*Mixture of cashews and almonds*
LUNCH	*Mackerel and green salad with garlic, oil and lemon*
DINNER	*Sturgeon, sword fish or tuna sautéed in butter Corn on the cob*
SNACK	*Corn chips*

BREAKFAST	*Small piece honeydew melon or watermelon 1 banana*
LUNCH	*3 ricecakes with cashew butter*
DINNER	*½ roast duckling with baked potato and steamed courgettes*
SNACK	*Popcorn*

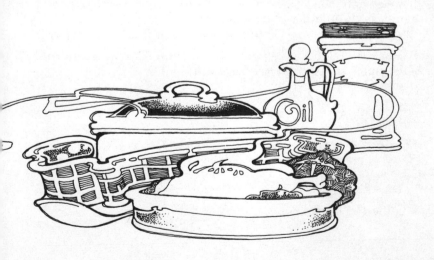

Food Recipes

BREAKFAST AND SNACKS

CANDIDA BREAD
(Phil Gernhard)

125 g/ 5 oz brown rice flour
2 eggs
150 g/6 oz grated carrots or
banana
150 g/6 oz safflower oil or
butter
1 tsp baking soda

1 tsp baking powder
¼ tsp nutmeg
¼ tsp cinnamon
½ tsp vanilla or other extract
3 tbsp yoghurt

Mix ingredients together in a bowl

Bake in a preheated 325°F/160°C (Gas mark 3) oven for 1 hour.

BANANA RICE BREAD

225 g/8 oz brown rice flour
50 g/ 2 oz corn flour
3 tsp baking powder
¼ tsp sea salt (optional)

100 g/4 oz melted butter
150 g/6 oz mashed bananas
225 g/9 oz corn syrup
2 eggs

Stir flour, baking powder and salt together.

In a separate bowl, beat the butter and corn syrup together, add eggs, beat and add the bananas; beat well then add the dry mixture; mix well. Pour into a small well-greased loaf tin.

Bake at 350°F/180°C (Gas Mark 4) for about 30 minutes or until a toothpick stuck in the centre, comes out dry. Do not overbake.

CORN BREAD

175 g/6 oz corn flour
50 g/2 oz brown rice flour
3 tsp baking powder
¼ tsp sea salt (optional)

3 tbsp corn syrup
240 ml/8 fl oz goat's milk or
soya
milk
3 tbsp vegetable oil

Mix the dry ingredients together.

In a separate bowl, beat the liquids together; add the dry mixture to the liquid, mix well. Pour into a small well-greased baking dish. Bake at 350°F/180°C (Gas Mark 4) for 25-30 minutes or until a toothpick stuck in the centre comes out dry. Do not overbake.

NON-YEAST RICE CARROT BREAD

275 g/10 oz brown rice flour
1/4 tsp salt (optional)
3 tsp baking powder
1 level tsp baking soda
2 eggs
3 tbsp honey

5 tbsp lemon juice
25 g/1 oz chopped carrots
25 g/1 oz walnuts, crushed
100 g/4 oz raisins
100 g/6 oz butter or margarine

Mix the dry ingredients together in a bowl.

In a blender, add the butter, eggs and milk. With blender running, add the carrots slowly until blended. Pour into a separate bowl, then add the walnuts, raisins and lemon juice. Mix well. Add the remaining dry ingredients and mix well.

Pour into a well-greased baking dish; tap dish on work top 2 or 3 times to settle mixture, set into oven at 350°F/180°C (Gas Mark 4). Bake for 25 to 30 minutes or until a thin sharp knife inserted in the centre comes out dry. Do not overbake.

RICE PANCAKES

1 egg
240 ml/8 fl oz goat's milk
2 tbsp sunflower seed oil
100 g/4 oz rice flour

1 tsp baking powder
1/2 tsp baking soda
1/2 tsp salt (optional)

Beat egg, add remaining ingredients in order listed and beat with rotary beater until smooth. Heat griddle greasing if necessary. To test griddle, sprinkle with few drops of water. If bubbles skitter around, heat is just right.

Pour batter from tip of large spoon or from jar onto hot griddle. Turn pancakes as soon as they are puffed and full of bubbles but before bubbles break. Cook both sides until golden brown.

BROWN RICE DELIGHT

100 g/4 oz mixed rices,
  including
long grain brown rice,
short grain brown rice,
basmati rice, and
other aromatic brown rices,
  according to availability

Paprika
Lemon pepper
50 g/2 oz French beans
50 g/2 oz beansprouts

Cook mixed rices in boiling salted water. Top and tail the French beans and slice diagonally; add them to the boiling water with the rice. Add immediately 3 dashes of paprika and 2 dashes of lemon pepper and cook the rice for about 20 minutes in all or until it is ready. At the end, when the rice is almost ready, stir in the beansprouts and cook for 5 more minutes. Serves 2.

BROWN RICE VARIATION

100 g/4 oz mixed brown rices
2 medium carrots, grated
50 g/2 oz raisins
1 tsp tarragon
Pepper

Cook mixed rices with tarragon and pepper to taste in boiling salted water. After 10 minutes, add grated carrots. After 15 minutes, add raisins, stirring gently. Continue cooking until rice is done.

BREAKFAST DELIGHT

1 papaya
1 kiwi
1 banana
Juice of ½ a lime
Raisins

Cut the papaya in half and scoop out the seeds with a spoon. Sprinkle with the juice of half a lime. Peel the banana and kiwi, cut in small slices and use to fill the 2 papaya halves. Serve cold. If liked, fresh berries such as raspberries or bilberries can be used instead of the kiwi fruit.

GARLIC CHICKEN

½ chicken
½ lemon
Garlic powder

Cayenne pepper
3 cloves garlic
2 tbsp olive oil

Place chicken in a baking pan and spoon over olive oil to cover. Squeeze the juice of the half lemon over the chicken, then sprinkle with a little garlic powder and cayenne pepper. Peel and crush the garlic cloves and add them to the pan. Place chicken in a preheated 350°F/180°C (Gas Mark 4) oven and cook for 25-30 minutes or until done. Serves 2-3 depending on size of chicken.

SALMON STEAKS

2 salmon steaks
Pinch of dill or thyme
4 cloves garlic

2 tbsp unsalted butter
1 lemon
2 tbsp olive oil

Melt unsalted butter in a pan. Squeeze the juice of the lemon into the melted butter. Peel and crush the garlic cloves and add them to the mixture of lemon and butter. Sprinkle the thyme or dill into the sauce:

Gently fry the fish steaks in olive oil, turning and basting with approximately half of the prepared lemon and butter sauce. Serve coated with the remainder of the sauce. Serves 2.

VEGETARIAN OMELETTE

3 large eggs
2 courgettes, chopped and diced
1 medium tomato, chopped and
  diced
1 tbsp parsley, finely chopped

Paprika
Lemon pepper
30 g/1 oz butter or 1 tbsp olive
  oil

In a bowl, beat the eggs with the courgettes, tomato, parsley and seasonings. Melt the butter or heat the oil in an omelette pan, pour in the egg mixture and cook for 5 minutes on each side until lightly golden.

Alternatively, cook for 5 minutes until the omelette is set and place under a hot grill to cook the top. Serve without folding.

BUCKWHEAT

1.2l/2 pints water   *200 g/8 oz unroasted buckwheat*
⅛ to ¼ tsp sea salt

Place the water and salt in a large saucepan and bring to a boil. While water is heating, place buckwheat in a wok or frying pan and toast over a high flame, stirring constantly, until it turns an amber colour and emits a deep aroma.

When the water is boiling add the buckwheat gradually to prevent the water bubbling over the pot.

Reduce the heat to low, cover and allow to simmer until water is absorbed (15-20 minutes). Remove from heat and allow to rest for 5 to 10 minutes. Using a damp wooden spoon, gently mix the grain from top to bottom while still in the pot. Cover again and allow to stand for 5 to 10 minutes before serving.

THE ULTIMATE DRINK
(*Betty Endicott*)

Papaya (1 large size glass)
Yolk of 1 free-range egg
1 banana
100 g/4 oz tofu, cut small
25 g/1 oz brown rice

Put all the ingredients together in a blender and mix to enjoy this thick, nutritious drink.

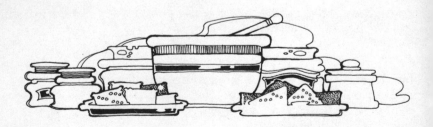

CARROT MUFFINS

100 g/4 oz rice flour
1½ tsp baking powder
1 egg

12 ml/4 fl oz fresh carrot juice
1 carrot, grated
2½ tbsp butter, melted

Preheat oven to 400°F/200°C (Gas Mark 6). Mix together flour and baking powder.

Beat egg, add juice, carrot and butter. Pour into flour mixture. Stir until just mixed but still somewhat lumpy.

Divide batter evenly into 8 muffin cups or bun tins, ½ full. Bake for 30 minutes.

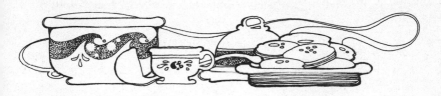

LUNCH AND DINNER

LEMON BUTTER SAUCE

75 g/3 oz butter
Dash pepper, to taste

3 tbsp lemon juice
2 tbsp finely chopped parsley

Melt butter in small saucepan over low heat. Add pepper, lemon juice and parsley. Cook until everything is well-heated. Serve at once. Makes about ½ cup sauce.

ASPARAGUS

3 tbsp olive oil
1 onion, thinly sliced
*½ green pepper, deseeded and
   chopped*
*500 g/18 oz can tomatoes,
   drained (but reserve liquid)*

50 g/2 oz chopped celery
3 tbsp juice from tomatoes
25 g/1 oz chopped parsley
Salt and pepper, to taste
450 g/1 lb fresh asparagus

Heat oil in large saucepan. Sauté the onion and green pepper until tender. Add tomatoes, tomato juice, celery, parsley and salt and pepper. Add asparagus and cook until tender. Serves 5-6.

SWEET POTATO JUMBLE

| 450 g/1 lb sweet potatoes | 3 tbsp miso |
| 1 tbsp sesame seeds | 3 tbsp stock |

Peel the sweet potatoes and cut in ½ inch dice. Steam or simmer until just tender. Set aside.

Heat the sesame seeds in a non-stick pan until they begin to jump. Remove from the pan immediately. Crush or grind in a food processor while still hot.*

Mix the crushed seeds with the miso and stock. Stir in the potatoes.

Using a non-stick pan if possible, cook over low heat about 5 minutes to blend the flavours.

Serve hot or cold as a side dish or rice topping. Serves 4.

Suggestions: Garnish with finely chopped spring onion, toasted sesame seeds or both.

*Or use a ridged Japanese grinding bowl called a suribachi.

EASY SOUP

450 g/1 lb sliced vegetables, such as onions, red pepper, tomatoes, corn, celery, spinach, marrow
2 tbsp finely chopped parsley
1.2l/2 pints good vegetable or chicken broth (look for canned or packaged bouillon in natural food stores, or make your own)
2 tbsp light miso blended with 4 tbsp hot water
Herbal salt and pepper, to taste
1 cooked potato, chopped in small pieces

Combine the ingredients and seasoning with the liquid, bring to the boil and simmer gently until cooked.

VEGETABLE STIR FRY

½ onion, chopped
2 stalks celery, thinly sliced
½ head cauliflower, chopped
½ head broccoli, chopped
1 carrot, pared into curls
1 green pepper, chopped
  (or thinly sliced)

225 g/8 oz mange tout
100-225 g/4-8 oz fresh
  mushrooms, sliced
Dash low sodium soy sauce
Dash fresh ginger, grated
1-2 cloves garlic, finely minced
2 tbsp oil

Wash and prepare all vegetables. Heat oil in pan. Sauté onion, garlic, celery, cauliflower, broccoli and green pepper. When still crisp, add carrot curls, mange tout, fresh mushrooms, soy sauce and ginger. Continue to cook until all vegetables are cooked through but still crisp. Serve at once. Serves 3-4.

WINTER LENTIL SOUP

100 g/4 oz lentils
350 ml/12 fl oz cup water
1 medium potato
1 small turnip
1 small carrot
1 medium diced onion
1 clove crushed garlic
¼ tsp thyme
3 tbsp soy sauce
Salt and pepper, to taste

Cook lentils in water, covered, for 25-30 minutes until tender but not mushy.

Meanwhile, dice potato, turnip and carrot (unpeeled if they are organically grown). Put them in a pot with water to cover, cook about 10 minutes or until just tender.

Add lentils and their cooking water, if any, to the vegetables. Add the other ingredients and simmer to make a fairly thick soup.

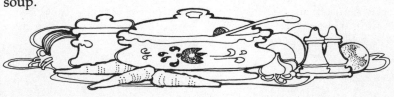

SEA STEAKS WITH ALMONDS

4 medium sized fish fillets
1 tbsp oil
1 tbsp butter
4 large spring onions, chopped

50 g/2 oz sliced fresh almonds
4 tbsp lemon juice
4 tbsp Worcestershire sauce
Freshly ground pepper
Dash cayenne

Wash fish and dry thoroughly. Heat oil and butter in pan; when hot fry the fish until brown on one side. Turn and cook on the other side. When fish is almost done, add spring onions. Cook a few minutes, then add mushrooms and cook a few minutes more.

Season with lemon juice, Worcestershire sauce, freshly ground pepper and a dash of cayenne. Serve hot. Serves 4.

BEAN AND LENTIL STEW

50 g/2 oz haricot beans, soaked
    overnight and drained
2 l/4½ pints water
100 g/4 oz lentils, rinsed
4 tbsp olive oil
2 medium-sized onions,
    chopped
4 cloves garlic, crushed
1 chilli pepper, finely chopped

25 g/1 oz rice, rinsed
1 tsp cumin
1 tsp oregano
1 tsp salt
½ tsp pepper
3 tbsp finely chopped fresh
    coriander leaves

In a saucepan, place the beans and water and bring to a boil, then cover and cook over medium heat for 1¼ hours. Add the lentils and cook for a further 20 minutes. In the meantime, in a frying pan, heat the oil, then sauté the onions until golden brown.

Add the garlic and chilli pepper, and stir-fry for an additional 3 minutes.

Add the frying pan contents and the remaining ingredients (except the coriander leaves) to the lentils and beans, then cover and simmer over low heat for 30 minutes or until the lentils and beans are cooked. Stir once in a while to make sure the stew does not stick to the bottom of the pot. Stir in the coriander leaves and serve hot. Serve 6 to 8.

LENTILS WITH SPINACH

4 tbsp butter
100 g/4 oz rice, rinsed
1.75l/3 pints boiling water
1 tsp salt
100 g/4 oz lentils, rinsed
4 tbsp olive oil
275 g/10 oz fresh spinach,
  thoroughly washed and
  chopped

4 cloves garlic, crushed
25 g/1 oz finely chopped fresh
  coriander leaves
½ tsp pepper
½ tsp cumin
1 tsp oregano

In a frying pan, melt the butter, then stir-fry the rice over high heat for 3 minutes.

Add 2 cups of the water and bring to a boil, then stir in ½ teaspoon of the salt. Cover and turn the heat to low.

Cook for 15 minutes, then turn the heat off and allow to cook in its own steam for 20 minutes. Set aside.

In the meantime, in a saucepan, place the lentils and the remaining 4 cups of water and bring to a boil. Cover and cook over medium heat for 30 minutes or until the lentils are cooked but not mushy. Drain and set aside.

In another frying pan, heat the oil. Add the spinach and garlic and sauté over medium heat until the spinach wilts.

Add the lentils, remaining salt, coriander leaves, pepper, cumin and oregano, then sauté for a further 8 minutes, stirring occasionally.

Place the frying pan contents on a flat serving dish, then spread the rice evenly over the top.
Serve hot. Serves 8 to 10.

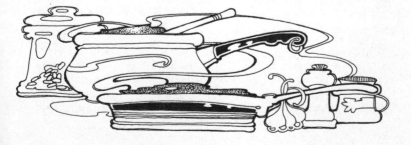

PEPPERS WITH BASIL

4 tbsp olive or vegetable oil
1 medium-sized onion, chopped
2 cloves garlic, crushed
4 large red peppers, seeded and
  chopped
1 tsp oregano

½ tsp sea salt
¼ tsp pepper
4 tbsp finely chopped fresh basil
  or tsp dried
2 tbsp lemon juice

In a frying pan, heat the oil, then stir-fry the onion and garlic until the onion turns limp.

Stir in the pepper pieces, oregano, salt and pepper, then sauté over medium heat for about 15 minutes or until the pepper pieces soften, stirring occasionally.

Stir in the basil and lemon juice. Serve immediately. Serve 4.

HERBED FISH AND RICE

2 tbsp oil
200 g/8 oz frozen peas
100 g/4 oz brown rice
4 medium cod fillets
3 tbsp chopped onion
Lemon juice
Salt and pepper

Paprika
2 tbsp salt-free Italian herb
  seasoning
250 ml/8 fl oz chicken broth
1 tbsp butter
475 ml/16 fl oz water
½ tsp curry powder
3 tbsp fresh parsley, chopped

In a medium sized saucepan, heat the oil and cook the rice and onion in it for a few minutes to toast the rice. Add the salt and pepper, the herb seasoning and the water. Bring water to a boil, turn to a low heat and cook 45 minutes until all water is absorbed. Cool. Add the chopped fresh parsley.

Refrigerate until needed. Oil a large casserole dish. Rinse frozen peas in lukewarm water and drain. Fill the casserole dish with alternate layers of peas and rice. Wash fish fillets and season with lemon juice, salt and pepper.

Arrange on top of the rice, sprinkle with paprika, dot with butter and garnish with strips of lemon peel. Mix chicken broth with curry powder. Pour around sides of casserole. Cover casserole and bake at 350°F/180°C (Gas Mark 4) for 30 minutes, covered. Uncover and bake a further 10 minutes.

TOFU STIR FRY

1 onion or 2 leeks (sliced)
2-3 cloves garlic (minced)
225 g/8 oz tofu (drained and cubed)

Put in a wok and sauté in 1 tablespoon sesame oil, adding a little more to prevent sticking.

ADD:

carrot and parsnip spears
broccoli florets and sliced stems
Chinese cabbage
chopped parsley
chicken broth or stock
salt and pepper
½ - 1 tsp arrowroot or corn flour (dissolved in water)

Vegetables should be tender but still crisp. Serve with brown rice or other grain.

ALTERNATIVE VEGETABLES:

cauliflower
courgette
bok choy (Chinese cabbage)
celery
green or red pepper
spinach

water chestnuts
beans or peas, sprouted
mange tout
celery
stoned and sliced black olives
toasted sesame seeds

VEGETABLE CHOP SUEY

3 tbsp sesame oil
175 g/6 oz shredded cabbage
50 g/2 oz sliced celery
50 g/2 oz sprouted peas
OR 100 g/4 oz frozen
  mange tout
100 g/4 oz bean sprouts

175 ml/6 fl oz chicken stock
1 tbsp arrowroot
25 g/1 oz toasted slivered
  almonds
1 red pepper, cut in 2 inch strips

Heat oil in wok and add vegetables. Fry 2-3 minutes over medium heat, stirring frequently. Add ⅓ of the stock. Cover and simmer 4 minutes. Mix arrowroot with remaining stock and stir into vegetables. Cook 2 minutes or until sauce thickens. Serve over rice. Top with almonds.

LAMB CHOPS WITH BASIL SAUCE

2 tbsp olive oil
8 lamb chops
1 tsp salt
1 tsp thyme
¼ tsp pepper
⅛ cayenne

1 medium-sized onion, finely
  chopped
2 cloves garlic, crushed
1½ tbsp flour
250 ml/8 fl oz water
2 tbsp dried basil, or 2 tbsp
  fresh, chopped

In a frying pan, heat the oil, then add the lamb chops and sprinkle with thyme, pepper, cayenne and ½ teaspoon of the salt.

Sauté over medium heat, turning the chops over a few times until they are well done. Remove the chops and place on a serving platter.

If there is too much fat in the frying pan, remove a little, then add the onion and garlic and sauté until the onion pieces turn golden brown.

Add the flour and stir-fry for 2 minutes, then stir in the water and remaining ½ teaspoon of salt. Simmer for about 2 minutes, stirring all the time.

Stir in the basil, then pour sauce evenly over the chops and serve immediately with mashed potatoes. Serves 4.

IMITATION CRAB, 'CREAMED' OVER RICE

2 tbsp butter
2 tbsp rice flour
250 ml/8 fl oz soya milk or goat's milk
½ green pepper, chopped
40 g/1½ oz parsley, chopped
225-450 g/½-1 lb imitation crab flakes
salt and pepper

Melt butter over low heat. Stir in rice flour then add soya or goat's milk, stirring to prevent lumps forming. Continue stirring until sauce thickens then add seasoning to taste. Add chopped pepper and parsley and cook for a further 5 minutes. Add crab flakes and cook, stirring gently, for 2-3 minutes. Serve over brown rice or other grain.

'CRABBY' VEGETABLES

50 g/2 oz butter
2 spring onions, chopped
2 garlic cloves, minced or finely chopped
275 g/10 oz fresh or frozen vegetables, cut up into even-sized pieces
225 g/8 oz imitation crab flakes
2 tbsp fresh lemon juice

Melt butter over low heat, sauté onions and garlic then add vegetables, crab and seasoning to taste. Cover and cook gently for 10 minutes or until vegetables are tender but crisp. Finally add lemon juice and serve with brown rice or millet. Alternatively, serve with Japanese buckwheat noodles or rice noodles.

CAULIFLOWER CASSEROLE

1 medium cauliflower
3 tbsp butter
3 tbsp rice flour
350 ml/12 fl oz milk or goat's
milk
½ tsp salt
⅛ tsp pepper

50 g/2 oz fresh parsley
(chopped) or
1 tsp parsley flakes (optional)
3 hard boiled eggs (thinly sliced)
50 g/2 oz crushed corn flakes or
tortilla chips OR brown rice,
OR crushed crispy cereal
2 tbsp melted butter

Separate washed cauliflower into florets and steam for a few minutes until tender but still quite firm.

Meanwhile, melt 3 tablespoons butter in saucepan. Stir in rice flour; add soya milk and cook, stirring constantly, until thickened. Remove from heat and stir in seasoning and parsley.

Layer cauliflower, sliced eggs and sauce into a greased casserole. Toss crumbs in melted butter. Sprinkle on top. Bake, covered, in a 350°F/180°C (Gas Mark 4) oven for 25 minutes. Serves 4-6.

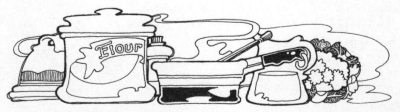

GOURMET BEANS

1 kg/2 lbs fresh green beans
1 tbsp sea salt
2.25l/4 pints boiling water
3 tbsp butter

2 tbsp lemon juice
2 tbsp minced fresh parsley
½ tsp salt, or to taste
⅛ tsp pepper, or to taste

Snap or cut off ends of beans. Just before cooking, wash quickly under warm water. Add beans and sea salt to water. Bring quickly to boil and cook, uncovered, until tender but still crisp (10-15 minutes), depending on the age of the bean.

Drain beans into colander. To serve, immediately melt butter in large pan. Add drained beans and stir until hot. Remove from heat; add lemon juice, parsley and seasoning. Stir.

Note: You can cook beans early in the day if you like. Drain and pour immediately into very cold water to cool quickly (this stops cooking and helps them stay crisp). Drain, cover and refrigerate. Later reheat and season. 8 servings.

RATATOUILLE

3 tbsp oil
½ medium onion, thinly sliced
1 large green pepper, cut in strips
1 medium courgette, thinly sliced
½ large (or 2 small) aubergines, diced
4-5 medium tomatoes, cut in chunks OR 1 450 g/16 oz can
    tomatoes
¾ - 1 tsp salt
¼ tsp ground white pepper
Dash cayenne pepper
Dash marjoram leaves (fresh or dried)
2 cloves garlic, minced
2-4 tbsp fresh, chopped parsley

Heat olive oil in saucepan. Add onion and green pepper. Sauté for a few minutes until onion is wilted. Add rest of ingredients. Mix well and simmer over low heat 15-20 minutes, stirring occasionally, until vegetables are just done.

Serve over rice (brown or basmati). 4-5 servings.

BAKED SALMON

1 half or whole salmon (2-3 kg/4 to 6 lbs)
100 g/4 oz butter plus 12 small pieces of butter to insert in slashes
25 g/1 oz flour (of choice)
75 g/3 oz chopped celery
75 g/3 oz chopped onion
1 large 800 g/1¾ can tomatoes (sugar-free)
2 bay leaves
paprika

Cut slashes in each side of the fish and insert the small pieces of butter. Place salmon on a large enough piece of heavy duty foil to wrap it for baking. Melt the rest of the butter in a saucepan. Stir in flour and brown slightly. Add chopped celery and onion. Then, add tomatoes and bay leaves. Season to taste with salt, pepper and paprika. Cook, stirring constantly, until sauce is slightly thickened. Pour the sauce inside and over the fish. Wrap foil securely around fish and bake at 325°F/170°C (Gas Mark 3), for 15 minutes per pound. Serves 6 to 8.

NON-DAIRY CREAM OF VEGETABLE SOUP

4 tbsp oil
50 g/ 2 oz rice flour
1.2l/2 pints water
¼ tsp sea salt
2 onions, sliced
3 stalks celery, sliced OR 100 g/4 oz vegetable of choice, chopped, eg broccoli
White pepper, to taste
Optional: add garlic and sauté with onion and vegetables

Heat 2 tablespoons oil in large saucepan; add rice flour and sauté. Cool and add water and salt, then simmer for 30 minutes. Heat a small pan. Add 1 tablespoon oil, onions, garlic if used, and vegetables, and sauté. Add them to the soup. Simmer 15 minutes more. Add pepper and chopped parsley if liked. Serves 4.

TOFU 'CHEESE' SAUCE

2-3 spring onions
2-3 cloves garlic
1 tbsp corn oil
225 g/8 oz tofu, drained and
    steamed
Fresh herb of choice, (eg basil
    or dill) Optional: carrots, red
    pepper, extra onion.

4 umeboshi (Japanese pickled
    plums, pits removed) or 4 tsp
    umeboshi paste
½ inch slice nuka (pickled
radish)
1 tbsp miso

Sauté onion and garlic in oil until slightly brown. Add any other vegetables and cook for a few minutes longer. Process or blend steamed tofu and all other ingredients until smooth. Use the sauce as a filling for omelettes or casseroles, or thin with water and serve hot over Japanese buckwheat noodles.

TOFUNAISE

225 g/8 oz tofu
1-2 cloves garlic, minced
Fresh dill, minced or dried dill

1 tbsp miso OR sea salt
1 tbsp fresh lemon juice

While food processor is running, drop in garlic and fresh herbs to mince. Add rest of ingredients and blend until smooth. Variation: try curry instead of dill to season.

May be used as a dip for chips or vegetables, as well as a substitute for mayonnaise.

SQUASH CASSEROLE

2 small or 1 large marrow or
    butternut squash
50 g/2 oz butter
½ - 1 tsp salt (according to
taste)
⅛ tsp pepper

1 tsp onion (minced)
3 eggs (well beaten)
25 g/1 oz crispy brown rice
cereal
    OR crushed tortilla chips
    OR crushed corn flakes OR
    crushed ricecake

Earlier in the day, cut butternut squash in ½ and scoop out seeds. Place, cut side down, on edged baking sheet. Bake 45 minutes-1 hour at 325°F/160°C (Gas Mark 3), until soft to the touch. Cool and peel.

In a food processor, mince the onion. Add eggs and process until well beaten. Add peeled, cooked squash and process until smooth. Add 3 tablespoons butter (melted), seasoning and a little soya milk (if desired). Pour into a greased casserole dish. Use remaining tablespoon of butter to top with buttered brown rice crispies or crumbs of your choice. Set dish in a pan of warm water and bake at 350°F/180°C (Gas Mark 4) until knife inserted in centre comes out clean (45 minutes - 1 hour). Makes 6 servings.

SPRINGTIME SPINACH

650 g/1 lb fresh spinach,
    washed
½ - 1 tsp salt (sprinkled) on
    spinach
50 g/2 oz butter
100 g/4 oz diced or shredded
    beetroot
2 tbsp lemon juice

½ tsp salt
⅛ tsp pepper
1 tbsp chopped fresh parsley
    (optional)
2-4 hard boiled eggs (yolks and
    whites divided)

Wash spinach, sprinkle with salt and cook in water that clings to leaves in a heavy saucepan, covered, for 10 minutes. Drain and chop coarsely. Heat butter in pan; add beetroot and heat thoroughly (If raw beets are used, first cook for 20 minutes in a covered pan with 1 tbsp oil before adding to butter.) Add rest of ingredients except egg yolks. Mash yolks and sprinkle on top. Makes 4-5 servings.

STEAMED VEGETABLES

1½ to 2 lb mixed vegetables (cauliflower florets, broccoli florets, sliced carrot, courgette and yellow squash)
100 g/4 oz butter
3 cloves garlic, minced

2 tbsp chopped parsley
¼ tsp oregano (optional)
Salt, pepper

Place vegetables on rack in steamer and steam over boiling water until tender but still crisp, about 15 minutes or less. Meanwhile, heat butter, add garlic and parsley and sauté lightly. Stir in oregano and season to taste with salt and pepper. Pour some of butter mixture over each serving of vegetables. Makes 6 to 8 servings.

PANACHE OF POTATOES A LA DUCHESSE

3 medium potatoes
3 medium yams
2 egg yolks

50 g/2 oz butter, melted
Dash nutmeg
Salt, pepper

Peel and quarter potatoes and yams. Cook potatoes in boiling water for 10 minutes or until done. Cook yams in boiling water for about 25 minutes or until done. Drain thoroughly and allow to dry slightly. Put potatoes and yams through sieve or ricing disc of food mill and blend well. Beat in egg yolks, butter and nutmeg. Season to taste with salt and pepper. Using pastry bag fitted with large fluted tube, pipe swirls of mixture around main dish on serving platter. Makes 10 to 12 servings.

IMITATION CRAB-VEGETABLE SOUP

2l/4½ pints chicken broth, imitation chicken broth, OR instant broth mix (yeast-free)

450 g/1 lb imitation crab flakes
1 small head Chinese leaves
  (cut up)
1 large or 2 small courgettes,
  sliced in thin rounds
Salt to taste

White pepper, a few shakes
Sesame oil, a few drops
2 spring onions, chopped
  (reserve some green top
  pieces for garnish)

Heat all ingredients to boiling. If desired, add few drops of sesame oil. Sprinkle with green onion tops or chives for garnish.

BUTTERY GRATED CARROTS

1 kg/2 lbs carrots
1 tbsp oil
¼ tsp finely chopped garlic

½ tsp salt
⅛ tsp pepper
50 g/2 oz butter

Pare or scrub carrots; grate or shred into large pan with tight fitting lid. Toss with oil, garlic, salt and pepper, and 2 tablespoons water. Cook, covered, over medium heat, stirring occasionally, for 10-12 minutes, or until tender. Remove from heat. Toss with butter to coat. Serves 4-6.

BUTTERY GRATED BEETROOTS

Use 1 kg/2 lb beetroot or carrots. Proceed as previous recipe, but cook beetroot for 20 minutes or until tender. Remove from heat. Toss lightly with butter and 1-2 tbsp lemon juice (adjust to taste). 4-6 servings.

BUTTERY GRATED TURNIPS

Use 1-5 kg/3 lb white turnips instead of carrots. Proceed as above, but cook turnips 15 minutes or until tender. Then to evaporate liquid, cook, uncovered, over very low heat for 5 minutes. Remove from heat. Toss with butter, 1-2 tbsp lemon juice, 25 g/1 oz chopped parsley - until turnips are coated. 4-6 servings.

LEMON BROCCOLI

1 kg/2 lb broccoli	*Juice of ½ lemon*
2 cloves garlic, halved	*Salt, pepper*
2 tbsp oil	*Lemon slices*

Split thick broccoli stems length ways and steam over boiling water until barely tender. Drain and cut into large pieces.

Sauté garlic in oil until garlic just begins to brown. Discard garlic and add broccoli to seasoned oil. Cook until tender, turning pieces frequently. Sprinkle with lemon juice. Season to taste with salt and pepper. Serve with lemon slices. Make 8 servings.

MILLET VEGETABLE SOUP

2 onions, finely chopped	*Sea salt*
¼ cabbage head, finely chopped	*1 bay leaf*
2l/3½ pints water	*Pinch of thyme*
100 g/4 oz millet	*1 tbsp miso or to taste*
2 diced carrots	*Finely chopped coriander*

Roast the millet and put in boiling water with all the vegetables, except the last three ingredients. Lower the heat to simmer, for 30 minutes. Keep pot covered while cooking. When ready, include last three ingredients, first dissolving the miso in some of the soup. Serve hot or cold.

BEAN SOUP

1 cup haricot beans	*1 teaspoon oil*
1-2 strips komb or wakame	*Miso or sea salt to taste* OR
2-3 large leeks	*Fresh or dried herbs (basil or dill*
1 onion	*goes well with this dish)*
2-3 bay leaves (optional)	*1 carrot*

Wash and soak haricot beans 7-8 hours. Drain. Bring to a boil in 1-2 litres (2 pints) water, with sea vegetable and bay leaves for one hour, covered, or pressure cook 40 minutes.

Slice leeks in half lengthways and wash well to remove all dirt; slice finely. Dice onion.

Sauté onion and leek over medium heat until soft and transparent—10-15 minutes.

When the beans are soft, add to sautéed leeks. Simmer 20-30 minutes over low heat. Purée some of the beans to give soup a creamy consistency, adding a little water if you want a thinner soup.

Chop fresh herbs (basil or dill) and add with miso and/or salt. Blanch carrot matchsticks for garnish.

AVOCADO DRESSING

2 tbsp oil	*Dash pepper*
1 large ripe avocado	*Dash cayenne*
3 tbsp lemon juice	*Optional: dash garlic powder*
¼ - ½ tsp salt (to taste)	

Mash avocado with fork; put ingredients in a jar and shake to combine or put everything into a blender or food processor and blend until smooth. Makes ¼ litre (8 fl oz) dressing

SESAME SALAD DRESSING

6 tbsp vegetable oil	*½ tsp sea salt*
25 g/1 oz toasted sesame seeds	*Optional: 100 g/4 oz chopped*
2 tbsp fresh lemon juice	*parsley*

Process in blender until nearly smooth. Refrigerate.

FRESH HERB BUTTER

1 spring onion OR ½ small
onion
   AND/OR 2 cloves garlic
   (chopped)
25 g/1 oz tarragon, basil,
   parsley, OR coriander leaves
¼ tsp salt

1 tsp lemon juice
¼ tsp white pepper
Dash cayenne
100 g/4 oz unsalted butter,
   softened

With food processor running, process onion and/or garlic until minced. Add herbs and salt and process until chopped (20 seconds). Add rest of ingredients and process until well mixed. Use as is, or transfer to wax paper or plastic wrap; roll into 1 by 8 inch cylinder. Freeze until ready to use.

TOMATO BUTTER

1 spring onion OR ½ small
onion
   AND/OR 2 cloves garlic
¼ tbsp fresh tomatoes

1 tsp lemon juice
¼ tsp white pepper
Dash cayenne
100 g/4 oz unsalted butter,
   softened

Process as in recipe above. Use immediately or freeze.

LEMON-SESAME SAUCE
(For asparagus or broccoli)

50 g/2 oz butter
Juice of ½ lemon
1 tbsp toasted sesame seeds
10 drops liquid sweetener

¼ tsp garlic salt
Optional: a little grated lemon
   peel

Melt butter and add lemon juice (and peel, if desired), sesame seeds and garlic salt. Stir and heat. Remove from heat and add sweetener.

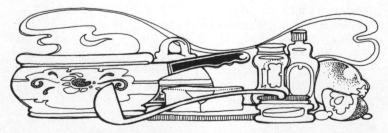

SPECIAL DIETARY SUGGESTIONS

As well as paying attention to what you eat and how you cook it, it is also important to observe some simple rules during meals or when shopping for food and planning menus.

- Chew food thoroughly 20 times each mouthful. Digestion begins in the mouth with the enzymes in your saliva.
- Drink liquids between meals, not with meals; liquids during meals will dilute the digestive juices.
- Eat less and chew well when emotionally upset since the digestive chemistry is changed, preventing complete digestion.
- Avoid overcooking since vitamins, enzymes and some proteins are all heat sensitive.
- It is best to eat small portions more often than large portions less often, since the spleen will aid the digestion of smaller amounts more easily.
- Avoid foods to which you are allergic; at the same time, avoid eating and drinking the same thing two days in a row. Exceptions are brown rice and water.
- Avoid distractions such as TV, radio, reading or driving while eating since you will not focus on chewing thoroughly and maintaining the relaxed mental state which assists digestion and assimilation.
- Read labels and ingredients on boxed, canned and packaged foods. When dining out, ask questions about the ingredients used in the food you are ordering.
- Keep a brief food-related-symptoms journal of everything you eat or drink to learn more about foods and how they affect your health. Record them over a period of time and review the records regularly.
- Do not eat protein with starches and fruits or starches with fruits. Ideally, eat tropical fruits by themselves, as a breakfast. Do not combine honeydew melon (or other melons) with any other food.

Your willingness to improve the quality of your life through healthier food choices and meal planning is a very significant step towards better health. Your willingness and action will produce the desired result. Following a healthy diet will make you more aware of the 'garbage' people eat. You will be stimulated to do better and acquire the energy, the body, health, mental and physical powers that you always dreamed of.

The area of greatest misunderstanding and confusion in the field of nutrition is the failure to properly understand and interpret the symptoms and changes that follow the beginning of a better nutritional programme. When we introduce foods of higher quality in place of lower quality ones, we have to understand the sudden onset of new, and not always improved, symptoms.

This is exactly what happens to Candida patients when they switch from regular junk food or food rich in yeast, to a protein-rich quality diet. The closer the food comes to the natural state, the higher the quality. Nuts and seeds, eaten in their natural state (unsalted and raw), are superior to chicken which, in its turn, is superior to beef. The quality of a nutritional programme is also improved by omitting toxic substances such as coffee, tea, chocolate, tobacco and salt.

A few important rules have to be taken into consideration by the patient who wants to recover from illness through a high quality diet. There is no doubt that the higher the quality of food we eat, the quicker we recover from disease, provided, of course, we are able to digest and assimilate the food properly. Proper food combining, proper order of eating the different kinds of food (the most easily digested food first), consuming the correct quantity and the correct time of eating (when hungry and not by the clock), should be cornerstone in our new eating habits.

Will following these rules bring us joy, a state of well-being and relaxation? Not quite. At least not immediately. The body still has to discard lower-grade materials and make room for these improved superior ones. Every cell in our body has amazing intelligence and aims always for improvement for better health, even though we seem to do all we can to interfere with this process.

What are the signs that become evident when we start to omit the lower-grade foods and instead, introduce superior foods? Toxic stimulants and lower-quality foods, where salt and spices have been added, have one thing in common: they are more stimulating than nut and vegetable proteins. Consequently, without them there will be a slower heart rate and initial letdown that lasts about 10 days and is followed by an increase in strength; this initial period is the regeneration period. Many patients stop their diet during this phase because they "feel better on the junk diet" and the new one makes them feel weak. In this regeneration phase, there is a shunting of energy from the exterior to the interior, or from the skin and muscles to the internal organs. Of course, this temporary muscle weakness is felt as a decrease in energy, since all the energy available is required to build up or balance the internal organs. In this crucial phase, it is very clear that the patient will have to rest more and restrict manual labour and sporting activities. This can also be restricting to the patient in his profession, and may require a leave of absence which in extreme cases could result in loss of employment. Success in recovery of health hinges upon the correct understanding of this point—realizing that the body is using its main energies in the most important internal work. So it is important to coast along in one's social obligations to a certain extent until this period is over.

As the food quality is raised, interesting symptoms start to appear. The body starts to remove the garbage, all the gross body obstructions. Wastes are certainly more rapidly discarded, then new tissue is made from the new, improved food. This becomes evident as weight loss. This is very clear in the case of the Candida patient: if they follow the anti-yeast diet well, they will lose weight. Lack of weight loss is due either to non-compliance with the diet or bad elimination of the garbage deposited in the tissues. Some patients are worried because of the continuous weight loss (although most are elated to finally lose some weight), but mostly this phase will be followed by a stabilization. Here, the weight remains stable and discarded material equals the amount of tissue formed by the more vital food. Finally, due to the improved absorption and assimilation, there will be an anabolic (rebuilding) stage but with minimal weight gain and increased energy.

One of the symptoms that occurs on a cleansing diet, such as the anti-Candida one, upsets many female patients. Often, there are skin eruptions and boils, especially on the face. Failure to understand this symptom may lead to a catastrophe. Lots of doctors will diagnose these skin rashes as allergies and prescribe the devil's advocate, a cortisone cream. They may not understand that this process is a favourable prognosis, well-known in acupuncture: the toxins are brought from the interior to the exterior. Discarding these toxins saves you from more serious diseases, especially degenerative ones. Often, the Candida patient has 'colds' with the coughing up of phlegm and may even have low-grade fevers. The biggest mistake we can make is to try to arrest these symptoms with medications, since the symptoms are part of a curing process. It is obvious at this point that patients who have had junk diets for most of their lives will manifest more of these unpleasant, but temporary, symptoms than people who have eaten better foods throughout their lives. So be happy when you observe these signs and realize that your body becomes healthier with each day that passes. Visualize this whole process as waste leaving your body, therefore, unable to bring further pain and havoc.

Some patients also believe that once their health is on the upward path to improvement, perfection is just around the corner. Alas, health returns in cycles; after a better diet, you have good days alternating with shorter times of negative symptoms. Also, do not forget that following a 'clean' diet will make you more sensitive to 'garbage' food. Before, you may have felt lousy all the time. Now that you have reached peak energy, sugar, for instance, may wipe you out for a day. Be glad your body does not allow you to eat inferior food any more. Nature has given you a second chance through purer diet and natural foods. Sit back and enjoy what happens: you can experience what it really is to feel healthy and fully alive!

QUESTIONS AND ANSWERS

Some questions always seem to come up. This is neither unusual nor surprising. Candida patients all go through the same struggle, but support is rare if not absent. It does not surprise me either that most of the questions are about diet: "When do I stop this 'boring' diet?", "When can I add some sugar?", "When can I have some wine or other alcoholic drinks?", and many more.

Let me first tell you that I am not happy with the term 'diet'. It has a temporary ring to it and sounds rather rigid. Most of us live to eat instead of eat to live. Unfortunately, much of our social life is incorporated around food intake which does not make it easier for the consumer who does not eat the 'regular' diet. But eating properly for your particular needs is simply a common sense 'way of life'. Certainly hunger has little to do with most of our eating patterns, but this most of us have yet to learn. I remember as a child my grandfather giving me candy and ice cream as treats almost daily. When I ended up being sick, the amount of those 'goodies' was even increased; no-one realised that the excess sugar in the first place was responsible for my trouble. And of course birthday parties, Hallowe'en parties, or any happy event seemed to be linked to sugar intake.

No small wonder that we become hooked at an early age! So often we adults are trying to fill an emotional void and it becomes a bottomless pit. We sit down to eat and do not even want to stop. The action of 'shovelling the food in' is to fill that bottomless hole which, of course, can never be filled by eating. Eating will only perpetuate it. Oddly enough, although this has been a lifetime habit, we only seem to become aware of it when we make changes in our diet.

Many people, after they start the change of eating, instantly feel better, stronger, less tired and do not experience any discomfort at all. Others, on the other hand, do experience various changes and within a few days many questions will arise.

How do I deal with sugar or bread cravings?

If you understand that the body desires the very food that it is cleansing from the system, it will make it easier to resist. Many times a craving means you are allergic to those foods you are craving or in the case of Candida patients, yeast cells seem to 'scream' for a particular food. You can easily visualize that the yeast cells make you crave those foods, there is a virtual war going on between your body and the Candida. The answer is to say NO to yeast foods! As the yeast cells decrease in number (through starvation and medications), the cravings decrease rapidly. It also helps to have some acupuncture treatments since there are points that can be stimulated for the relief of cravings.

I ate something wrong, does this mean I have to start all over again with my diet and medications?

No! I get many frantic calls from people in despair because they have "gone off their diet". Not only do they feel uncomfortable physically but they feel quite wretched mentally. Often, the guilt feeling can become even more negative than the incorrect food. I think it is important for the doctor and the patient not to be too judgmental. I tell my patients that I hope they enjoyed that food (which usually is not the case) but even more important, I hope that they monitored their reactions to the intake of yeast foods. When we break our diet, we should observe what is happening, gain understanding, and go back to our correct way of eating. As time goes on, 'cheating' seems to happen a lot less because we feel better and do not want to return to those physical and emotional lows associated with junk food. Most of us have the habit of eating too much too fast and we are not likely to change these habits overnight. In the beginning, we have the tendency to eat huge quantities of new 'allowed' foods, but eventually we will level off. There should come a time when we eat only a fraction of what we used to eat and can even go on a day of fasting with vegetable juices. When I mention this to some patients, they shake their heads in disbelief and try to convince me that they will have no energy. How surprising it is when they discover that they have a lot more energy!

I am feeling tired, even more than usual.

This is absolutely normal at the beginning of your new diet. A decrease in energy is a particular problem during the first two days. This is nothing but a cleansing process and you need all your energy to eliminate the toxins. This is obviously not the time for strenuous labour, sporting events or competition. Rest more, go to bed on time and realize that this period will soon pass. Do not commit the mistake of eating more or, even worse, of giving up on the new diet, since you felt a lot 'better' on the old one. The same reaction happens again when we start taking anti-fungal medications. Due to the die-off of the Candida organisms and the production of Candida toxins, the body feels sluggish until you are able to eliminate these poisons.

I am feeling deprived and depressed: food is uniformly dull.

In the early days of your diet, it is not the time to wine and dine. You will find it increasingly difficult to have lunch at your favourite restaurants. Looking at your friends and family devouring everything you can not without any consequences (at least none that are immediately visible), is rather depressing. You feel punished and isolated. All these new foods seem tasteless. However, I can assure you that you will grow to love these foods so much that it would not occur to you to want to change. You feel more and more energetic with every bite of this diet, a feeling you have missed for years. Hang in there and you will see that your period of feeling deprived should not last longer than two weeks.

When may I start adding new items to my diet or re-introduce some of the foods I was eating in the past?

It is wise to stay as closely as possible to the outlined diet at least for the first month and possibly for two months. At that time it is wise to introduce new foods one by one and to monitor your reactions closely. If your body is not ready to consume these foods, you will immediately (within the hour), experience fatigue, headaches, bloating or other yeast-related symptoms. Do not view this as a negative reaction but be grateful that you are more in tune with your body. It warns you immediately when 'toxic' substances are introduced. Try those same foods again at a later date. The ideal situation for all of us is to really know what the body needs and can handle. This is health! It is a learning process for all of us, and is one that we all must discover for ourselves.

I am not satisfied; I am hungry all of the time, even immediately after eating.

It is that addiction again, that same old habit of stuffing yourself full of food whenever something goes wrong or becomes difficult. It happens to almost everyone in these early days. Eat some 'allowed' snacks (nuts and seeds), eat more frequent, smaller meals and only when you feel up to it, do some moderate exercise. The feeling of being hungry immediately after your meals is related to the presence of Dampness and Heat in your Stomach-Spleen area. Look at your tongue and you will see a white-yellow coating in the middle of it. Acupuncture treatments can assist you in draining this Heat-Dampness from your body.

I am used to having coffee; do you recommend any substitutes?

It is amazing that many patients think they cannot start their day without the energy boost of coffee or sugar. This is what I would like to call 'false' energy. Yes, indeed, you might feel some pick-up after this cup of coffee but for sure you will crash down an hour later unless you repeat the intake of these stimulants. You do not need that early morning coffee to 'get you going'. It is like flogging a dead horse! You will soon be aware of how much you cheated yourself and mother nature for all those years. It is a beautiful discovery to feel what true energy is like once you get over the initial stage of addiction and withdrawal.

What happens when I travel, when I visit friends or when friends visit me?

When you travel, do the very best you can. It is amazing to see that people removed from the daily stress and from the normal environment with fog, dampness or cold, seem to be able to cheat more easily without suffering all the consequences. It tells you right there how much our immune system can suffer from environmental and emotional factors. When you take a trip, you are off to have fun and to relax, so please do not be too uptight about being good about your food intake. You always can find fish, vegetables, grains or turkey and you can request a restaurant to grill fish, steam vegetables and cook brown rice.

Visiting friends should not be too much of a problem. Read the chapter about coping with Candida, and you will know how to get help from your friends to stay 'straight'. Real friends will be happy to cook what you like out of respect for your habits.

When people visit you, there should be no problems at all! Your guests will be surprised that healthy cooking is equal to delicious cooking. No uncomfortable feelings such as flatulence or distension, should occur and at the same time, you should feel total satisfaction after each intake of your new diet.

Why can my friends eat whatever they want and stay healthy?

One man's food is another man's poison. We all have these differences: other people might be genetically less susceptible, have better control over their emotions or live in a better environment so that the negative food factor has a smaller impact. But do not always believe what you see. You have no way of knowing how your friends feel after their junk food intake. You will not see that they cannot fall asleep because of distension, gas or stomach pains. You have no way of knowing that they are constipated or susceptible to mood swings and depression. Besides, this matters little. You are in there for yourself, for achievement of your better health and longevity. When your friends are ready, they too will make the switch.

Chapter 3

Anti-Fungal Therapies

KILL THE CANDIDA

After being the victims of medications for such a long time, most Candida patients are not very enthusiastic about returning to any medication at all. This is understandable. However, as I already stressed before, as an enemy, Candida is a tough one! It took clever advantage of your weakened immune system in order to invade your body. In their turn, the yeast cells will continue to suppress your very important defence mechanisms. And this is where the anti-yeast medication comes into play: its role is to break this vicious cycle. But it is important to realize that medication intake alone will not do the job. This part of the treatment is the easiest: we already live in a world sensitized to medication intake. Again, we have to stress the importance of all the steps of the treatment. The different anti-yeast medications are described in chronological order, with their advantages and disadvantages.

1 NYSTATIN POWDER

Numerous cases document the efficacy of the first drug of choice, Nystatin, in the treatment of Candida. A very small dose is taken to start with, only enough powder to cover the tip of a toothpick, and each day the dose is built up when tolerated.

Day 1: one toothpick
Day 2: two toothpicks
Day 3: three toothpicks when tolerated
Day 4: 1/8 tsp plus 2 toothpicks
Day 5: 1/8 tsp (x2) plus 1 toothpick
Day 6: 1/8 tsp (x3)
Day 7: 1/4 tsp plus 1/8 tsp twice a day
Day 8: 1/4 tsp twice a day and 1/8 tsp once a day
Day 9: 1/4 tsp three times a day

With a doctor's advice, the dose can be built up to a full teaspoon three times a day when tolerated. Mixed with a little water, Nystatin is easy to take. It can also be dissolved in water and added to an enema, providing a concentrated dose to the sigmoid and rectum. In cases of post-nasal drip, it is useful to sniff the powder (as directed), so that the drug is delivered directly to the nasal cavity, a mucous membrane that is fertile ground for Candida growth.

DISADVANTAGES?

A major disadvantage is that Nystatin is not a broad spectrum fungicide. While effective for certain strains of Candida, numerous, potentially pathogenic fungi are unaffected by it. Strains of Candida resistant to Nystatin have also been described. It is not unreasonable to assume that, as with antibacterial antibiotics, an increased use of Nystatin will eventually result in the emergence of Nystatin-resistant strains of Candida.

Nystatin is a mould by-product and may cause allergic reactions in the mould-sensitive patient. In my practice, up to fifty per cent of patients have this problem. It is also difficult to determine the correct individual dose since this is different from person to person. It is also difficult for the patient to distinguish adverse reactions from die-off symptoms, page 88. Some adverse reactions are nausea and vomiting, while withdrawal symptoms are usually noted when Nystatin intake in halted.

Although safe, these negative characteristics of Nystatin suggest the need for other agents which used synergistically can minimize the drawbacks, while maintaining or exceeding Nystatin's record of safety and efficacy.

In practice, I rarely prescribe it as a first line medication, but keep it in mind for resistant cases and local use.

2 KETOCONAZOLE TABLETS (NIZAROL, 200mg)

This is a potent anti-fungal drug. It is a synthetic broad spectrum anti-fungal agent available in white tablets, each containing 200 mg ketoconazole. Nizarol is easy to take since it requires only one tablet daily.

It is THE anti-fungal medication for the presence of Candida in the oesophagus. Patients with burning in the chest, and difficulties in swallowing should add this drug to their therapeutic regime. Nizarol requires an acid environment to be dissolved. In cases where antacid medications or H_2 blockers such as Tagamet are needed, these should be given at least two hours after Nizarol administration. Nizarol is also contraindicated in cases of pregnancy and breast feeding.

Nizarol is usually well tolerated. The most frequent adverse reactions are nausea and vomiting, which occur in 3% of patients. Cases of liver damage have also been reported and patients require careful repeat monitoring each time the drug is prescribed.

3 AMPHOTERICIN (Fungilin tablets, 100mg; Fungizone powder, 50mg)

Broad spectrum anti-fungal medications, preferable in some instances to Nystatin. Few adverse reactions have been reported to these drugs but side effects include temporary prolonging of the menstrual cycle; the cycle returns to normal when medication is stopped. Dose as prescribed.

4 CAPRYLLIC ACID (Caprystatin tablets, 100mg)

Caprystatin contains 100mg of Capryllic acid, an effective agent against Candida at least *in vitro* studies. Further studies have shown that it can be effective in the treatment of Candidiasis. Capryllic acid is a fatty acid and is thought to replace some of the fatty acids normally produced by intestinal bacteria when these have been disrupted by antibiotics or immunosuppressive drug treatment. It should be administered at least an hour before or after meals. If gastro-intestinal discomfort is noted, however, it may be taken during meals. Dosage: for the first week, one tablet, twice daily. For the second week, two tablets twice daily, followed by three tablets daily. Average duration of treatment is 2 to 3 months at the therapeutic dose followed by 4 to 6 months on a maintenance dose of two tablets daily. This particular preparation of Capryllic acid contains a relatively low dose of 100mg but this can be an advantage for allergic patients or those who suffer from severe die-off symptoms (page 88). Caprystatin is not advised during pregnancy.

5 CAPRYLLIC ACID (Capricin capsules, 300mg)

Many studies have been carried out to find out the form of Capryllic acid most effective in the treatment of Candida. The special coating of slow-release formulations appear to be more effective because they allow for a uniform release of Capryllic acid along the entire length of the gastro-intestinal tract. A therapeutic dose of twelve capsules, taken in two or three doses over the day (or as directed) should eliminate most of the Candida. Capricin should be taken for 16 days then a maintenance dose of two tablets twice a day should be taken for a further period of two months. It is important during that time to try to build up the immune system (page 93) so that recurrences are less likely. It is advisable to take this medication with food since some nausea can occur if it is taken on an empty stomach.

6 ANTI-FUNGAL HERBS

Both Red Clover and Yellow Dock have been found to be effective in the treatment of Candida since both have a mildly toxic effect on yeasts. Yellow Dock Root contains vitamins A and C as well as the minerals Manganese, Nickel and Iron. It has many medicinal uses and acts as a nutritional tonic.

7 BENEFICIAL BACTERIA

Replacing normal intestinal flora is one of the keys to the successful treatment of Candida. Bacterial supplements provide beneficial strains such as Lactobacillus acidophilus, Lactobacillus bulgaricus and Bifidobacteria, all of which are thought to help maintain a healthy intestinal flora. Specific directions for dosage should be followed and the advice of your doctor or pharmacist sought if in doubt.

8 GARLIC

The world has always been divided in two camps over garlic: those who love it and those who detest it. The first camp would include the Egyptian pharaohs who were entombed with clay and wood carvings of garlic and onions to ensure that meals in the afterlife would be well seasoned. It would include the Jews who wandered for many years in the Sinai wilderness, fondly remembering "the fish we eat in Egypt so freely, and the leeks, onions and garlic".

The camp of the onion and garlic haters would include the ancient Greeks, who considered the breath odour of garlic and onion eaters vulgar, and the Egyptian priests who "kept themselves clear from it . . .".

Chemists must be included among the garlic lovers. For them, the reasons are professional. In recent times, clinical experiments have confirmed most of those ancient ideas about garlic power. In fact, it appears that the healing powers of garlic may be far greater than previously anticipated.

Garlic has been literally on the breath of the physically fit for over 5000 years and is now being rediscovered all over again by the medical and scientific community. It has a long history of medicinal use. The Babylonians used it to treat disease as early as 3000 B.C. Garlic was the food of the slaves working on the Pyramids; it was said to give them strength to endure hard labour. The Greek athletes relied on garlic rather than an anabolic steroids for increased energy and stamina.

The Romans used garlic as a diuretic and worm expeller. Aristophanes believed that garlic juice could restore man's flagging virility. Hippocrates, the father of medicine, used garlic for a wide variety of ailments. Louis Pasteur, the great microbiologist, was a firm believer in garlic because of its anti-microbial and anti-bacterial activity. Albert Schweitzer used garlic in Africa for the treatment of dysentery and cholera.

Garlic was used as an antiseptic for the prevention of gangrene and septic poisoning during World Wars I and II and saved thousands of lives. The Soviet government has imported garlic from Europe to fight flu epidemic, at one time importing as much as 500 tons. At the turn of the last century, family doctors treated asthma, whooping cough, and tuberculosis with garlic and had excellent results. Garlic has been effective against several of the bacterial cultures resistant to commonly used antibiotics including penicillin. Attention to its anti-fungal powers was established when sufferers from a fungus-related inflammation of the brain, cryptococcal meningitis, were treated with garlic. Garlic alone, or garlic used with other drugs, was found to be 85% effective. Garlic extract acts as a potent anti-fungal and anti-bacterial and garlic's sulphur-containing compounds and minerals have other beneficial actions: S-allyl cysteine protects liver cells, Germanium and Selenium help to stimulate the body's immune response and the chemical allicin is known as Nature's antibiotic.

9 PAU D'ARCO TEA

Quickly gaining popularity in the treatment of Candida is the South American herb Pau D'Arco, which is often referred to by its other Spanish names: Ipe Roxa, Lapacho and Taheebo. It is currently hailed for its effects on cancer (in South America) and Candida.

Pau D'Arco consists of the inner bark of a large tree that flowers a vibrant pink, purple or yellow, depending on the species. Throughout South America, Pau D'Arco is used as a remedy for immune system-related problems, such as colds, fevers, infections or snake bites. It was one of the major healing herbs used by the Incas.

Toxicity of Pau D'Arco is very low. It may loosen the bowels, which is frequently desirable in the Candida patient. Up to three to four cups a day may be taken, while it is an excellent idea to use some of the tea together with Lactobacillus in an enema. Using an enema twice a week quickly brings relief of some of the die-off symptoms, especially 'brainfog'.

CONCISE TREATMENT PLAN

Week 1:

- The anti-yeast diet (page 32)
- Lactobacillus acidophilus preparations as directed
- Pau D'Arco tea, 2 cups daily (add cinnamon or lemon if desired)
- Garlic, 6 capsules three times a day with meals
- Biotin, 5mg daily

Weeks 2–4:

- Continue with the diet suggestions for Week 1 and add Capryllic acid (Capricin, 300mg) as follows:

Day 1: 1 capsule three times a day (with meals)
Note: if 2 meals only are taken, take 1–2 capsules (a total of 3) with each meal
Day 2: 2 capsules three times a day
Day 3–7: 3 capsules three times a day
Day 8–16: 4 capsules three times a day
Day 17 onwards: 2 capsules two times a day (maintenance dose)
Note: the maintenance dose can be continued for 1 month and if necessary for a further 2 months. Taking the medication for longer than this should not be necessary if you stick to the recommended diet plan.

Week 5:

- Continue on the maintenance dose of Capryllic acid (Capricin, 300mg)
- Continue with the diet suggestions for Week 1
- Start adding the following foods:
  - yeast-free rye or wheat breads (available from health food shops)
  - maple syrup or a little honey
  - fruits such as canteloupe, peaches (without skins) and berries
    Note: eat fruits separately from other foods, for example, for breakfast
- Boost your immune system by adding the following:
  - Vitamin C, 4000–10,000mg daily (depending on bowel tolerance)
  - Vitamin E, 400 IU daily
  - Selenium, 100mcg daily (or combined with Vitamin E)
  - Zinc orotate, 50mg daily
  - Evening Primrose Oil (each capsule 40mg GLA), 4 capsules daily

Note: from Week 1 onwards it may also be beneficial to have acupuncture treatments to increase the energy in the Spleen-Pancreas and boost the immune system. A suggested programme of treatment is: once a week for 4 weeks. From Week 5 onwards once every 14 days for 1 month, then once every 3 weeks for 2 months.

THE YEAST DIE-OFF PHENOMENON

When high doses of Capryllic acid are given, all of a sudden thousands of yeast cells will be killed. The dead toxins formed from these yeast cells will temporarily overwhelm the patient's organism, causing symptoms sometimes more uncomfortable than the symptoms of the disease itself. "I am not better, but worse" is a frequently heard complaint at the beginning of therapy. These die-off symptoms usually appear between the 2nd and 5th day of medication and will usually last for one week (sometimes two). After this period most of the Candida cells are dead and eliminated, so that fewer remain to be killed, limiting the amount of the die-off.

What are the Symptoms?

Any of the yeast-connected symptoms may surface during the die-off, especially flu-like symptoms, brain symptoms such as foggy thinking, concentration and memory decrease, muscle and joint pains, tightness in the chest with palpitations and even a feeling of irritation and a film over the eyes. It is not unfamiliar for a patient to state that they feel drunk and in a state of incapacity. Thinking about these symptoms, it is no wonder that some 50% of Candida patients have at sometime been admitted to a psychiatric ward.

How Do We Avoid or Alleviate the Die-off Symptoms?

Follow the anti-yeast diet as strictly as possible, especially during the first two weeks on an anti-yeast medication such as Capryllic acid. Remember that each time you cheat, you give the yeast cells a chance to grow.

Start taking the anti-yeast medication during the second week after your first visit to your doctor; during the first week you start with the diet, acupuncture, supplements (Acidophilus) and natural killers such as garlic and Pau D'Arco tea. These latter remedies will kill a lot of yeast cells, clearing the way for the Capryllic acid to do its work.

Do not start with the full dose of the medication but build up the dose gradually so that your body can adjust to the die-off.

If possible, try to take a break during the period you expect the heaviest die-off, or plan it during a weekend.

During the period when you have 'foggy brain' symptoms, drink a lot of water with lemon juice; this will help clear toxins.

Make sure you have regular bowel movements; toxins are eliminated via the stool.

To stimulate your whole system, use the brushing technique: take an ordinary (clean) clothes brush and brush as if you were cleaning your clothes. Brush the following areas starting at the lower inside of the leg, brush your way up to the groin; then brush downward starting with the outside of the thigh, all the way down to the ankle; continue on the outer side of the arm up from the wrist to the shoulder and then back down from the inside of the elbow to the wrist. What you are accomplishing with this is stimulating the energy meridians in the direction of the flow of energy through the body, relieving any stagnation and helping to eliminate toxins.

In spite of all this, many patients still go through extremely uncomfortable die-off symptoms, but once they get through it, the reward is great: it feels wonderful to be able to think straight for the first time in a long period and this will give you hope that there is a definite chance for improvement.

ELIMINATING TOXINS

One of the pillars in the successful treatment of Candida is the maintenance of a regular bowel movement. Constipation is almost always present in the case of Candida, inducing die-off symptoms. We frequently see what is referred to as a 'roller-coaster' phenomena: the patient feels excellent at 9 o'clock in the morning, two hours later, unexpectedly, they feel entirely different. This is due to the presence of toxins: at nine in the morning this patient's colon may be relatively free of toxins, but after breakfast and the first dose of medication, yeast cells are killed and toxins form. If the patient does not evacuate these toxins immediately, they will be overwhelmed. These sudden changes in behaviour do not always contribute to the acceptance of the disease by family members or friends.

I cannot list all the possible natural remedies that are available to ensure proper evacuation but a list of the ones that have proven to be effective in my practice follows.

Fibre in the diet

Dietary fibre is a broad term covering a complex mixture of many substances. Initially, it was defined as being the 'roughage' of plants, the part left over at the end of the digestive process. Grain fibres such as wheat or rice bran are largely insoluble. By absorbing water and swelling within the intestines, they help to reduce the bowel transit time, the time between intake and elimination.

Recent research into the beneficial aspects of fibre has centred around substances such as pectins, gums and mucilages found in many fruits, vegetables, oats and pulses. These form viscous solutions that soften the stool and may enhance nutrient uptake in the gastro-intestinal tract.

A key factor in the high fibre diet is rapid transit time from intake to elimination. Studies have shown that African children on their native diet have transit times of eight to twelve hours, while some elderly people may have transit times of up to fourteen days! The stool is made softer and bulkier by pectins and cereal fibre makes it easier for food to pass through the colon, inhibits the excessive growth of bacteria and, by causing the colon to stretch to handle the increased bulk, permits relatively fewer carcinogens to come into contact with the walls of the intestines. In some people, fibre may also help to inhibit the absorption of cholesterol.

Keeping to a well-balanced, low fat, high fibre diet makes it easier to lose weight since the greater bulkiness of high fibre foods causes most people to feel full and thus reduce their intake. And, of course, such a diet is usually low in calories.

Government dietary recommendations are that we should increase our intake to 30 grams of fibre a day, depending on our body weight (larger individuals should consume more). However, do not add too much fibre at once: it takes a few days for the system to adjust. In some people too much fibre can cause intestinal gas and discomfort and loose stools, symptoms that are already present in most Candida patients. Intake of water should also be increased – to six glasses a day – as an increase in fibre causes a need for more water in order to bulk up the stool. Also, be aware of the higher loss of trace elements and other important substances such as calcium, iron, zinc and magnesium that accompanies a sudden increase in fibre intake. The latter elements are extremely important for the Candida patient and any deficiency will trigger or maintain the growth of the yeast.

You can easily add fibre to your diet by increasing the amount of fruits, vegetables and nuts that you serve. Perhaps one of the easiest meals at which to increase fibre is breakfast. Rice bran, nuts and brown rice should be among the favourite breakfasts for Candida patients.

PREVENTING FURTHER SPREAD

We have discussed the spreading mechanism of Candida on page 12. In order for the Candida patient to avoid the spreading of yeast cells to the bloodstream, and thus giving the opportunity to the cells to invade almost all the organs, the interruption of this vicious cycle is an absolute priority. Biotin, taken at levels of at least 3mg will cut the transformation cycle from the yeast to the fungal form. This daily dose should be taken with the first dose of the anti-fungal therapy (page 82). We should not forget that Biotin is a B-vitamin, and may feed the fungus. However, the cutting of the vicious spreading cycle is more important at this point.

The amount of the Biotin is also important. Many multivitamin preparations contain it but usually at levels not above the microgram (mcg). This will not be enough for our purpose. The daily dose should be 3–5 mg. Biotin has been administered for prolonged periods at dosages as high as 40 mg a day without adverse effects. It is also one of many water soluble vitamins that can be depleted by stress. Biotin is essential in the conversion of carbohydrates to energy, and also plays a major role in the synthesis of fats and in protein metabolism. Other conditions known to be associated with lowered or deficient levels of Biotin are: loss of hair, anorexia, lassitude, muscle weakness, hypercholesterolaemia and depression.

REPLACING THE NATURAL FLORA

The composition of the normal gastro-intestinal flora is discussed on page 12. We know that the presence of these billions of friendly bacteria (Lactobacillus acidophilus and Bifidobacteria) are essential in order to inhibit the growth of yeast cells. Normal flora can be destroyed after only a few days of antibiotic use, for instance, and need to be replaced in order to avoid the creation of a favourable environment for the yeast. By supplementing your daily diet with stable, high potency L. acidophilus and Bifidobacteria preparations, you will greatly enhance your body's natural ability to keep pathogenic microorganisms under control. As an added bonus, daily supplementation of Lactobacilli products increases the absorption of nutrients, reduces blood cholesterol levels, maximizes the efficiency of the digestive system, and greatly enhances the immune system.

There is more to the make-up of the healthy microflora than Lactobacillus acidophilus. We have already mentioned Bifidobacteria, which is predominantly found in the gastro-intestinal systems of breast-fed infants. Around the age of seven years the balance of microflora changes from Bifidobacteria to Lactobacillus acidophilus, which then becomes the predominant strain in the gastro-intestinal tract. In approximately 5% of the population, this change does not take place, and we find that these particular people get more positive results from supplementation with Bifidobacteria.

Almost every Candida patient can benefit from taking Lactobacillus acidophilus; in so doing, they repopulate the gastro-intestinal tract with the indigenous form of friendly bacteria and, thus, improve the strength of their immune systems.

It is most beneficial for anyone who is just beginning their supplementation programme to begin by using both the acidophilus and the Bifidobacteria in order to obtain the maximum benefits. Depending on the type of diet that the person is accustomed to, the ratios of acidophilus to Bifidobacteria are as follows:

Lacto-vegetarians, Asians, and non-Western cultures: 80% Bifidobacteria and 20% L. acidophilus.

Individuals on standard Western diet: 80% L. acidophilus and 20% Bifidobacteria.

BOOSTING THE IMMUNE SYSTEM

As little as twenty years ago, the question of strengthening the immune system was not even considered. Now the answer to this question seems to be the best sought secret on our planet.

What can we have done to our immune systems to allow such diseases as AIDS, Leukaemia, Herpes Simplex, Systemic Candidiasis recurrent EBV (Epstein Barr), and CMV (Cytomegalovirus) to take their toll. These immunosuppressive diseases are reaching epidemic proportions and Systemic Candidiasis in terms of numbers can be put at the top of the list. We may take medications to kill the viruses or yeast; we may find out the source of contamination and, thus, control the spreading; we may find a nutritionally-oriented doctor and be put on an appropriate diet. Unfortunately, the anti-viral medications are not only deficient, they all have dramatic side effects. Surely the most logical method of combatting a disease is to PREVENT it in the first place.

Every minute of every day wars rage within our bodies. The combatants are so small that we do not even notice these battles. Our immune systems have evolved legions of defenders, specialized cells that silently rout the unseen enemy. Sometimes the penetration of our defences by these invaders is successful, however, and results in allergic reactions, colds, flu, yeast infections, or in extreme cases, AIDS.

The human immune system functions as a kind of biological democracy, wherein each member has a certain task. The defender white blood cells fall into three groups: the phagocytes, or 'cell eaters', and two kind of lymphocytes, the T and B cells. They have only one objective: to identify and destroy all cells that are not part of the human body.

How does the battle begin? As viruses invade the body, some are consumed by the macrophages (cell eaters). These are the frontline defenders, who then summon Helper T cells to the scene. The Helper T cells identify the enemy and begin to multiply. Helper T cells then recruit and activate Killer T cells who are specialized in killing cells that are infected by foreign organisms. A second class of defenders called to the war scene are the B cells, normally based in the spleen and lymph nodes. The Helper T cells activate the multiplication of these B cells which start forming antibodies.

Meanwhile, some of the viruses are successful enough to invade human cells. Killer T cells will simply sacrifice these cells by chemically puncturing their membranes or walls. The viruses released from those cells will be neutralized by the antibodies produced by the B cells, which will bind directly to the viral surfaces.

Once the infection is contained, Suppressor T cells halt the activities of the B and T cells, preventing them from going out of control. As an extra defence barrier, Memory T and B cells are left in our bloodstreams, ready to move in if the same viruses should ever invade our bodies again.

Of course, the enemy is sometimes very deceptive. Many viruses have found devious methods to escape early detection. Common cold viruses for example, constantly mutate, changing their 'finger prints' so that our bodies have to continually design new antibodies to combat them. Other viruses hide out in healthy cells or even worse, are able to kill Helper T cells, the commanders in chief of our immune system, thereby short-circuiting the whole defense mechanism.

1 SUBSTANCES TO AVOID:

As much as possible leave out of the diet noxious factors such as over-chemicalized foods and bleached flour. Avoid excessive smoking and drinking, chemotherapy and radiation. When you are subjected to the above agents, boost your immune system by taking the following measures.

2 SUPPLEMENTS:

a. ZINC: The thymus shrinks in size and function early in life. This results in a limited ability to produce T cells. By supplementing with zinc (Zinc orotate), 50 mg per day, the thymus is effectively bolstered even when supplements are begun late in life. Do not forget that zinc is deficient in many diets, particularly among the elderly who need it most. Since it is not uncommon for zinc tablets to cause stomach upset, they are best taken shortly after a meal. Natural sources of zinc are steak, lamb chops, pork, pumpkin seeds, eggs and mustard. Soya beans, turkey, most nuts, peas and berries also contain zinc. Zinc orotate seems to be exceptionally well-tolerated and absorbed and is a natural product. Zinc is best tolerated on a full stomach but better absorbed on an empty one. So it is a choice between the tolerance of the gastro-intestinal system versus absorbability. The supplement is especially indicated in young people suffering from recurrent colds, growth disturbances, flu and allergies, pregnant and lactating mothers and the elderly.

b. IRON: Iron is another mineral with positive effects on the production of T cells through its involvement with several bacteria killing enzymes. Systemic Candidiasis and Herpes Simplex infections are both conditions which are more prevalent with individuals who are iron-deficient. Natural sources of iron are pork liver, beef kidney, red meat, egg yolks, oysters, nuts, beans, asparagus and molasses

c. BETA CAROTENE: The precursor of Vitamin A, Beta carotene is recommended by the American Cancer Society. The advantage of taking this material over Vitamin A is that there is no danger of overdosing since Beta carotene is converted to Vitamin A only as needed. One capsule, 25,000 IU, daily is a sufficient dose. Natural sources are: mangoes, cabbage, spinach, carrots, greens and sweet potatoes.

d. SELENIUM: Selenium is yet another essential mineral which is associated with cancer prevention and a strengthened immune system. It is known to activate production of co-enzyme Q, which, in turn, stimulates the immune system. Deficiency of selenium causes a reduction in the number of lymphocytes and phagocytes, cells which consume foreign pathogens. A daily dose of 100 mcg is advised. Natural sources are bran, tuna, onions, tomatoes and broccoli.

e. VITAMIN C: A minimum daily allowance of 4000 mg Vitamin C is recommended, and if tolerated (absence of diarrhoea), up to 20,000 mg will boost the immune system. Natural sources are citrus fruits, berries, tomatoes, cauliflower, potatoes and sweet potatoes.

f. VITAMIN E: One vitamin stands out as essential in defending the body against environmental chemicals, and that is Vitamin E. It acts as a powerful anti-oxidant. In other words, it has the strongest ability to protect against chemical damage of the cell membrane. It is one of the most important factors in controlling blood pressure and protects against heart disease. This essential nutrient is easily destroyed by the oestrogens in birth control pills. Vitamin E is also believed to protect against certain forms of cancer, especially skin cancer. Since a woman taking the pill has little or no protection against cancer-causing agents activated by the UV rays of the sun, she has a slightly greater risk of developing skin cancer.

If that same patient is smoking and overweight, the danger of developing a blood clot is alarmingly high! Vitamin E is an anti-coagulant, important in preventing abnormal coagulation of the blood. Good sources of Vitamin E are cold-pressed oils, spinach and eggs. A recommended daily dose of Vitamin E as a supplement is 400 IU.

3 ACUPUNCTURE:

There are two ways of increasing the strength of our immune system. First of all, through acupuncture, we can increase the amount of defence energy in our body by stimulating certain points on the body meridians. People with recurrent colds, viral infections, and yeast infections are helped by increasing that kind of energy. The other way is even more important since it involves the stimulation of the spleen organ. This organ, besides its important role in the digestive function, also has a key role in the production of white blood cells and therefore a key role in our immune system. Through stimulation of spleen points, located on the meridians (pathways), the energy in the spleen organ increases and strengthens our immune system. A well-balanced person will rarely get sick. One of the theories in acupuncture, well accepted now, is that stimulating acupuncture points will release endorphins and enkephalins. Both substances are natural pain killers. They also seem to reduce anxiety and create a sense of well-being. Even more startling, some studies suggest that they affect macrophages and T cells, therefore enhancing the immune system.

4 DIET:

Cold food and raw food will adversely affect the spleen. The Candida diet is a good example of an immune boosting diet, although in the absence of Systemic Candidiasis more variety is allowed. Steamed vegetables, eggs, fish, chicken, turkey, sweet potatoes, potatoes, tropical fruits, bread (rye or wheat), soy sprouts, miso, lean meats (with a minimum consumption of beef), buckwheat, millet and oats, are all important substances in an immune boosting diet. Avoid any cold or raw foods since they will create 'Heat-Damp' in the spleen, decreasing the energy in that organ.

5 EMOTIONS:

Each organ is linked to certain emotions. The spleen (or our immune system) is related to worry and obsession. People with spleen deficiency are typical A-type personalities: analytical, intelligent, meticulous and fixed in the Freudian anal stage (extreme cleanliness, obsessive, compulsive personality). If you want to minimize insults to the immune system, you had better change this lifestyle!

6 EXERCISE:

Mens Sana in Corpore Sano (a healthy spirit in a healthy body) should be your life slogan. Exercise will move the energy in the meridians, bringing the body into better balance. Exercise may also result in increased levels of INTERLEUKIN 1 and INTERFERON, both of which strengthen our defences. When helper T cells encounter an enemy, they release a spurt of Interleukin which causes other lymphocytes to multiply so it follows that anything which enhances this immune response will be beneficial.

ANTI-CANDIDA SUPPLEMENTS

The most effective combination of supplements, especially when there are nutritional deficiencies accompanying the toxic or allergic manifestations of Candida are:
• Magnesium
• Essential Fatty Acids
• Vitamin B6

1 ABNORMAL METABOLISM OF FATTY ACIDS (EFA)

Only a few years ago, the role of Essential Fatty Acids, such as gamma linolenic acid (GLA), was largely ignored by researchers, medical practitioners and nutritionists. With the advent of the prostaglandins (PGs) and the discoveries which related their importance to good health, all that has changed. The key ingredient in Evening Primrose Oil, GLA, is effective in treating a diversity of ailments, including acne, arthritis, PMS, overweight conditions, hypertension and a host of other health problems.

Perhaps even more importantly primrose oil appears to be one of the most potent agents of preventive medicine of all time. Throughout most of its history, the whole plant has been used as a herb and in 1919 in Germany, two chemists reported the presence of unusual fatty acids which they named GLA. It was not until the sixties that scientists discovered the high biological potency of the oil. In 1982 the Nobel Prize for Medicine was awarded to the three researchers instrumental in the discovery of the prostaglandins (PGs), whose importance to good health is difficult to overstate. These essential fatty acids are the precursor of the PGs. They are called essential because they cannot be made by the body and must be provided ready-made in the diet. Two essential fatty acids, Linoleic Acid and Linolenic Acid are required for proper membrane structure and function of all body cells.

Provided there is enough linoleic acid in the diet and the metabolic processes are functioning normally, the body can use linoleic acid to produce GLA. Unfortunately, a number of facts can prevent this reaction from happening. Among the culprits are: sugar, cholesterol, saturated fats, consumption of alcohol, diabetes, aging and viral infections. Common nutritional deficiencies such as in Zinc, Magnesium and Vitamin C, can also slow the reaction.

Fortunately, by supplementing the diet with the GLA in Evening Primrose Oil, harmful affects can be eliminated. A dose of 40 mgs GLA four to six times a day will be of help in combatting most of the above mentioned health conditions.

2 MAGNESIUM

Magnesium seems to get less of the attention that other minerals receive. However, it is vitally important to our body as it performs many functions. There is now evidence that sudden heart failures among young men are possibly due to a lack of this mineral. A balance of magnesium and calcium in the body is known to promote the smooth contraction of muscle, including the heart.

Magnesium and calcium work together (we need twice as

much calcium as we do magnesium), but in high doses these two minerals can act antagonistically.

Deficiency of magnesium results in many disorders: irritability, anxiety, depression, muscle tremor, muscle twitches and convulsions. Where does this deficiency come from? Intake of diuretics is one major cause. Several of them tend to produce marked drops in levels of magnesium. Excessive alcohol consumption is another reason. The diet of elderly people is often poor in magnesium and, of course, they are the ones that most commonly take diuretics.

3 VITAMIN B6

This important vitamin helps the body assimilate proteins and fats. It prevents various nerve and skin disorders and works as a natural diuretic and muscle pain reliever. Natural sources for the Candida patient are: liver, kidney, heart, cabbage, eggs and beef. In supplement form, 50 mg daily is a sufficient dose.

4 OTHER NUTRIENT DEFICIENCIES

The most common deficiency of the Candida patient is a low level of iron as measured by serum iron levels. Iron deficiency is a known predisposing factor to Candida infection, so these low levels should be taken seriously.

Other noted deficiencies are Folate deficiency, Vitamin A (with normal serum carotene), Vitamin C, B12, and Biotin deficiency. Correction of these low levels will reduce the growth of yeast cells.

Another important factor is the synergism or teamwork between proteins and Vitamin A. The body cannot utilize protein without Vitamin A. Without sufficient amounts of Vitamin A, protein cannot be stored in the major depot, the liver. This vitamin also seems to be essential in changing the protein we eat into the protein which becomes part of body tissue.

Calcium intake is another necessity, especially for women during the menopause. With a low-intake of dairy products, the intake of calcium is minimal. But there is another reason: high protein diets, such as the Candida diet, may disrupt your calcium balance. Augment your protein intake to 150 grams a day and you will lose considerable precious calcium in your urine. It is therefore a good idea to increase your intake of calcium (and phosphorus) substantially while you are on a high protein diet for any length of time. The recommended dose of calcium is 1500 mg (2 tablets of 750 mg) taken at night.

QUESTIONS AND ANSWERS

How do we know we are better or how do we measure the improvements?

Does this question surprise you? I have heard it in practice so often. It is normal human nature to forget bad times and to feel only the present. I have often to recall to patients what the original symptoms were like because they tend to focus on the actual problems of now, sometimes magnifying them. Of course, with the occurrence of strange 'healing' symptoms, the patient can get confused. Are these healing, die-off, or Candida symptoms, is another frequently heard question.

There are several methods to measure improvement after treatment. The easiest one is to look at all the symptoms involved. It is advisable to fill in a questionnaire similar to the self-scoring diagnostic test on page 20. Even after one month, patients are surprised when they repeat this questionnaire and see that many of the symptoms have either disappeared or lessened in degree. There is otherwise no way for the patient to remember how they felt about a particular disturbance in the body.

Another objective sign of improvement is the tongue picture. Looking at the tongue has always been a meaningful diagnostic test but has fallen into disgrace because of all the modern laboratory tests available. However, you can hardly find a more objective sign of your health. For an acupuncturist, it is one of the most important diagnostical steps. What is a normal tongue picture and what do we see with the Candida patient?

Ideally, tongue picture diagnosis should be performed in bright sunlight, in order to avoid false interpretations. Tongue diagnosis gives important and objective information, and gross changes can be distinguished easily. A normal tongue, found in a healthy individual, is neither engorged (fat) nor constricted (thin). It has a moderately red colour, is relatively wet and has no coating (fur) or at most a thin, white coating. The tongue is divided into areas which correspond to the different organs. The area important for the yeast patient is the middle part of the tongue. View the tongue in the morning before eating, it will constantly change during the day, under the influence of food intake.

The tongue shows different signs with the Candida patient. We see in the middle area of the tongue a white, sometimes yellow coating. The thicker the coating and the more yellow the colour, the graver the disease. It is a definite sign of improvement when the yellow colour changes to white and the coating thins.

How long do I continue with the medication?

This is one of the most difficult questions to answer. Each patient can be in a different stage of the condition and be subject to different triggering factors. Most of the recent research on anti-fungal drugs, however, indicates that there is a tendency to underdose and to misjudge the length of therapy. It is a fact that most patients relapse about three months after stopping the therapy, mainly because not enough was done during treatment to boost the immune system. For medications, follow the dosage regime suggested in the earlier part of the chapter.

With Capryllic acid once you are on the maintenance dose of two capsules twice a day, keep to this dosage for 14 days. During this period carefully monitor your reactions. If many of the yeast symptoms come back in spite of the maintenance of a good diet, increase the intake to four capsules three times a day for at least another fourteen days. Then, try to go back on the maintenance dose.

What is the relationship of Candida with EBV (Epstein Barr Virus), CMV (Cytomegalovirus) and MVP (Mitral Valve Prolapse)?

From experience, I have seen that a high percentage of Candida patients also suffer from EBV and CMV. This should not come as such a surprise. You get Candida because of a suppressed immune system. Therefore, viruses such as EBV can slip more readily through your defences. The virus remains in your B cells and becomes reactivated at moments of decreased resistance.

A correlation between MVP and Candida also seems to exist. Not much research has been done on this subject but for the most part the condition remains stable and patients can lead a normal life.

Chapter 4
Candida: The Psychological Aspects

PSYCHOLOGICAL PROFILE

Feelings of frustration and of being misunderstood and rejected seem to be part of our life experience. To a Candida patient, these feelings are often magnified; life seldom seems to treat the Candida patient fairly.

In the early childhood experience of the Candida patient, abuse often has been present. The experience of sexual, emotional, or physical abuse are indications of a traumatic childhood, in which emotional nourishment, encouragement in goal-setting, or simply the coherence of a healthily functioning family are absent.

This fear-inducing environment influences the immune system, weakening it and leaving one susceptible to invasion by diseases. Ancient medical practices, such as acupuncture and homoeopathy, have indicated the relationship between physical illness and the emotions. According to the philosophy of acupuncture, each emotion is linked to a certain organ. Fear, for instance, will decrease the energy in the Kidney organ, worry and pensiveness will do the same in the Spleen. A sudden, extreme shift in one's emotions will thus affect one's equilibrium, leaving one temporarily open to the invasion of viruses, bacteria, yeast cells, or in the worst case, to the onset of debilitating disease. A good example is the occurrence of rheumatoid arthritis after a sudden, extreme fearful event: a divorce, sudden death in the family or loss of a job are all situations related to extreme anxiety and fear. This negative emotion will deplete the energy in the Kidney organ, and usually leads to the onset of the first arthritis attack a couple of months later. What makes it even worse is that deficiency of energy in the Kidney organ leads to more fear and anxiety, pulling the patient in a vicious circle.

What fear does to the Kidney, worry does to the Spleen. People become obsessed with the past, isolate themselves, leading to a crash down of energy in the Spleen.

What follows next is the common nightmare of the Candida

patient. As children, most of these patients were given antibiotics and subjected to our modern diet with preservatives and sugars. Most of the symptoms will appear a couple of years later, but sometimes immediate yeast-related signs surface: mood swings, depression or suicidal tendencies. The sudden mood swings are the most startling symptoms. Patients look and act joyful at 10 am and are threatening to kill themselves by 2 pm. We can understand the scepticism and disbelief of professionals and family; nobody, not even the patient, expects these sudden variations. At the end, patients themselves are convinced that they have become crazy: it is the only possible answer to this yo yo behaviour.

You know where the real problem of the Candida patient starts? Most of these victims, especially in the beginning stages, look almost too healthy, too handsome . . . in fact, they look too good to have any kind of disease! This is the Catch-22: outwardly, it does not look like a disease. And, the text-book physician, looking for objective signs, hardly ever finds them. How can you see 'fogginess' in the brain, burning urination, severe PMS symptoms, decreased attention span. . . . At most, the patient looks depressed. 'Go shopping', 'treat yourself to a cake', (how ironic), 'take a short holiday', or other pieces of well meaning advice are frequently given.

The emotion that predominates in this disease, however, is ANGER! All Candida patients have a reservoir of anger, mostly deeply hidden. There is a need to understand the origin of anger and to seek means of dealing with the factors involved. Do not believe that this anger will always show in violent behaviour. There are other levels of manifestation of anger: ulcerative colitis, hypertension, eczema, migraine attacks, depression and suicidal tendencies can all be expressions of this emotion. Most patients will not even admit that they are angry. However, a lot of their expressions imply underlying anger. 'I am bitter about the way my doctor treats me' or 'I am fed up the way my husband denies this problem', 'It irritates me, I cannot get any explanation from anyone', are only anger in disguise. In fact, anger, frustration and irritability are all emotions linked in acupuncture to an imbalance in the Liver organ.

However, I feel that it makes more sense to recognize and accept the anger as such. Patients who find no place to put their anger are ridden by guilt, which offers no relief. Letting the anger out, little by little, is like relieving some steam. Somebody in a support group said, "Since nobody seems to understand my problem, I stopped talking about it". She might not be aware of it, but there is an immense amount of anger behind this passive behaviour.

Another manifestation of hidden anger in almost every Candida patient is their bodily reaction to it. An almost constant symptom in these patients is pain in the neck and shoulder region. We all know the expression, 'you are a pain in the neck', these patients actually *have* a pain in the neck because they are angry and they refuse to accept it or are not allowed or do not allow themselves to express the anger outwardly.

Of course, this chronic disease elicits anger from the rest of the family, especially the partner, as well as the patient. The patient may build up the anger for all kinds of reasons. They feel constantly rejected, are always questioned and doubted about the existence of the disease, and simply because they are outside the mainstream, they do not get their share of the world's excitement and rewards. The partner resents the disease immensely because it makes them a prisoner in their own house, without even having the disease. They are inconvenienced by their partner's illness and this leads to feelings of frustration and resentment.

Why do some of these patients turn out well, while others go completely on the wrong track, socially and healthwise? I believe that we use the frustrations of growing up to form a certain force that will be constructive for the first group, but destructive for the latter one. Candida patients, as a group belonging to the most abused ones, unfortunately use that energy to manifest their anger, isolating themselves and being labelled 'trouble makers', 'nuts', or 'lazy'. Crying spells in a Candida patient are nothing else but an expression of their anger and are, in fact, in a lot of cases, their sole outlet for it. At least crying may trigger more sympathy than overt hostility and irritability, but in essence, it will be the same. During their whole lives, anger has been built up so much that it needs only a small stimulus to erupt in a volcano of stored-up emotions, unfortunately, easily aimed at the wrong persons. Children have an easier time expressing their anger, directly towards the person involved. My son, at the ripe age of six, expresses his anger towards me very easily, "I hate you". It does not make him a monster, all he is saying is, "I am angry at you".

Returning to the Candida patients, their mood swings can turn into suicidal thoughts, the ultimate form of their bottled up anger, turned against the self. The anger and frustration can be so big, that they are literally 'trying to kill themselves', mainly as an expression of their anger and dejection, turned inward.

What can the patient do to channel this anger in a positive force? First, the patient has to accept that there is anger. It is my experience that most Candida patients do this. Their first sentence to me is often, "I am angry at all these doctors . . .". For them to identify the source of this emotion is not so difficult, at least not at first hand. Doctors who are not able to diagnose the disease are the main culprits for many lost years. I am sure some of these doctors deserve the anger they get for being narrow-minded and incompassionate. It is typical for abused children to feel guilty: they must have attracted this abuse because of their behaviour. However, since this anger had no outlet in childhood, the doctor-patient relationship is perfectly suited to let some steam off and to direct some anger at another person.

Of course, many Candida patients know exactly why they are angry. They have been wandering around for years, suffering with pain, depression, fatigue, but the person they turned to for help, their doctor, failed to recognize the source of their problems. Once patients realize it was not 'all in the head', and have lost, therefore, years of their lives, they naturally berate all those doctors for not supplying the help they needed.

How can we deal with this anger?

We might confront those doctors that failed to recognize our condition. However, in case of the Candida patient, it might be a Catch-22: even now, most doctors deny the existence of this disease, adding fuel to our anger. So, it might be necessary to find some other outlets for our emotions. Do not fall into the trap of becoming angry! Better communication with the direct family to create an immediate support group is a satisfactory solution. And, it is an excellent idea to take the spouse along to Candida support groups, to meet other people with the same problems.

Going through these different steps should really solve the problem. Unfortunately, life is a lot more complex, and theory does not always translate into practice. However, dealing better with your anger will avoid turning this negative feeling against yourself, hampering your full recovery. Drive, determination and a positive mental attitude will prevent breakdowns.

The real key to resolving most of the problems for any patient is good communication. That's what the next section is all about. Mark Fowler and Gloria Axelrod explore useful tips for the Candida patient to overcome most of the painful situations they are confronted with.

There is one more important psychological aspect of this disease: patients that are recovering, or even completely healed, have a hard time to let go of sickness and reach for new responsibilities and vitality. Friends will no longer need to support their weakness so they sometimes get less attention and sympathy. They may also lose some of their celebrity status, since Candidiasis is sometimes 'fashionable'. Some patients try to get by in spite of feeling OK, simply because it is too scary after all these years to face the real competitive, neurotic world. Patients have to take a solid stand to change, to move on with their lives and leave behind this old foe, Candida. I must say, though, that a very positive aspect of these patients is their willingness to help other people with the same condition. I have never seen a group more eager to help fellow sufferers overcome the different difficult barriers in their recovery. I guess this disease changes you forever!

COPING CONFIDENTLY WITH CANDIDA
(Contributed by Mark Fowler and Gloria Axelrod)

After several mornings of waking up tired, grumpy and apathetic, you decide that nothing is working out. You're not getting any better. Your allergies are acting up, you're not concentrating properly, you have less and less energy.

When you finally see the doctor, after rushing to get there and then having to wait, you explain your depressing condition. The doctor says there doesn't seem to be any justification for your unusual symptoms. He asks if they might be psychological in nature.

Though he phrases it nicely, it still boils down to 'your problems are all in your head'. Frustrated and disheartened, you realize this situation is life-threatening to you—but you wonder how you can make that clear to anyone else? It's often hard to get doctors' assistance for a disease they can't see or identify. Much easier to have a broken limb!

Frustrations of an Illness

Candida is not easily treatable because many of the symptoms are vague. Also, as discussed in the body of this book, the medical profession is only beginning to accept its full scope and impact.

You don't tend to group Candida with ominous life-threatening illnesses like heart disease, cancer, arthritis or AIDS. But any illness, even a headache, disrupts your life when it invades your own person. People needed to help—doctors, therapists, friends, lovers, family, bosses—want to participate, to come to the rescue. But they don't know how.

Communication is challenging because each person's frame of reference is different—and constantly changing. When you add unique Candida symptoms, the stress of illness, and the generally apathetic medical environment, the Candida sufferer is in an exceptionally difficult position.

Getting Help

Assume responsibility. The question is: how do you get help? The first step is to be responsible—ask for it. As one of Doctor De Schepper's patients said, "We have a responsibility. We got ourselves sick, we've got to get ourselves well. I had to go through three doctors before I found Luc".

When your health is at stake, you must take charge of guiding others to help you help yourself. A perfect example of the situation we are discussing occurred several years ago to Mark. It was not Candida-related, but it was definitely life-threatening.

Mark was visiting a woman friend for the first time, and was waiting for her to get ready to go out. He was sitting in the kitchen waiting, while her two teenagers were in the living room watching TV. They had only just been introduced. Eating some potato crisps, Mark accidentally inhaled a piece of crisp.

After several attempts to remove the crisp, he realized he could not breathe or speak. Fear was the first reaction: I don't know anyone here, how do I tell them what's going on, how much time do I have?

Realizing he truly needed help, he walked over to the teenage boys. Picking the closest boy, Jack, who seemed also the most friendly, he took Jack's hand, strongly but gently, looked into his eyes very seriously and mouthed silently, "I need your help".

He guided the boy up from the chair, and turned around. Mark then took Jack's hands and arms and put them around his chest. He motioned Jack to pull his hands hard into Mark's chest . . . the Heimlich Manoeuvre.

Jack did it, and it worked the first time! Mark could breathe again. He thanked Jack, hugged him, and went on to have a wonderful evening, glad to be alive.

Well, great story, but what does this have to do with Candida? Everything. Mark found that when he took responsibility to ask for someone's help, gently and calmly, he got it.

Asked later why he so easily responded to Mark's request, Jack said he knew Mark was serious and needed help. Jack felt he had no other choice but to respond.

Jack and Mark became partners—a team. Those of us with Candidiasis, Mark included, need teamwork and information. Mark had read about the Heimlich Menoeuvre, but was not trained in it. You may not be trained in any particular therapy, either, but you have your own symptoms, experiences, readings and discussions to draw on.

The two most important means of support for you as a Candida patient are a successful and satisfying working relationship with your doctor, and the reinforcement and understanding of those closest to you: your family, and friends.

While we primarily address doctor and family, giving you some techniques that will help, these same techniques can be used with waiters, waitresses, bosses and medical insurance personnel, as they are basically universal.

Probably one of the hardest things for all of us to do is receive help. "I can handle it, I don't need help", seems to be a big part of our personal philosophy. We are quick to help others, but slow to ask for it ourselves.

The key is: we are usually ready to help the other guy. Let's take advantage of that situation and give them the chance to be happy—by helping us. But, first we must make it clear we NEED help.

Let's take a situation common to all Candida patients who may have tried several therapies and 'cures' but still have the same symptoms and who don't seem to be getting well.

Working with your Doctor

When the initial treatment doesn't work, our first reaction might be to strike out at the doctor for not 'curing' us. It is here that a little preparation before you visit your doctor comes in handy.

Be Prepared
1. MAKE A LIST of exactly what you did since you last met the doctor. Did you follow your diet, any prescription, etc.? Did you notice any unusual symptoms or habit changes? Try to crystallize what happened so that you can give that information to the doctor. He is not a mind reader, and the only way he can help is to get all the information.

After you have made your lists, read them over to see if there is anything additional that might help. Next, outline what you want to talk to the doctor about, for example: goals, concerns, question or problems.

This may seem like a lot of work, but being prepared is critical to giving and receiving meaningful information. It also helps to relieve your anxiety and concern because these thoughts, questions, ideas, feelings are no longer swimming around in your head—they're down on paper!

Armed with your list, you can meet your doctor with added confidence.

2. Explain that you have all this information as soon as you meet with your doctor. (It would be appropriate to mention this when you telephone for your appointment but messages often get lost or garbled). Ask if he has the time to discuss it now. He might prefer to reschedule or suggest an alternative. Explain that this is not a routine follow-up, it is a major point in your therapy when you believe change is necessary. It is IMPORTANT to you, and your doctor needs to realize that.

3. State your overall objective and your concern about reaching it. It is important to keep it simple and to the point. The following paragraph might be your introduction: "Dr Smith, I seem to be feeling worse, and I'm experiencing some unusual symptoms. I'm very concerned about this, and about my therapy in general. I've made a list of my symptoms, questions and concerns. Do you have the time today to help me with it?"

You have stated your problem, that you're prepared to work together, and you're asking for help. The ball is in the doctor's court as to how he or she can help. You and the doctor can develop options TOGETHER as to how to handle the time scheduling.

Let's review the above suggestions:
1. Be prepared by making a list of concerns and goals;
2. Let other people know your objectives;
3. Solicit their help, and let them know you're in it together.

Three Sentence Rule

You don't want to bombard the listener with too much information. To help you with this, there is a technique we call 'the three sentence rule'. It can help you present information simply, clearly and, most importantly—with few words.

When you have so many things to say, it's hard not to say them all at once, especially at such an emotionally challenging time. If you can keep your communications to small digestible bits of information and wait for feedback, you have a better chance for success.

109

Not simple, you say. You're right—it does take practice. Fortunately, because we think faster than we talk, we have time to do some editing in our heads.

In the FIRST SENTENCE, state the subject you want to discuss. Next, ADD A SENTENCE that will start to clarify that subject. Third, ASK FOR FEEDBACK. You'll begin to get a feel for your listener's interest, and whether there's enough time to explore more deeply.

Take a minute to review the sample conversation with Dr Smith. As you go through the paragraph, you will notice that sentence one brings up the subject of unusual symptoms. The second sentence stresses that the symptoms and the therapy are a concern. The third sentence expands on the topic and asks the doctor whether there is time to discuss these concerns. It says a great deal in a short period of time.

This technique looks simple, but it takes time to get comfortable with it. Be patient with yourself. Give it time and practice. We have found that our students, just by trying the three sentences, become more clear and concise. By editing their material, they are encouraging their listeners to respond.

To review the Three-Sentence Rule:
1. Sentence one - state your subject;
2. Sentence two - say something about the subject;
3. Sentence three - ask for feedback.

ASKING CLARIFYING QUESTIONS AND LISTENING FOR THE ANSWERS

After you have presented your situation, wait and listen to what the doctor has to suggest. Your doctor might say, "I'll take whatever time is necessary to help now. You are a valued patient and I know this has been a difficult time for you".

On the other hand, they might just say "I've come to the conclusion that there's not much I can do. I'm as stumped as you are with your situation. I think I need to recommend another doctor for you". Whatever the response, it is vital that you take responsibility for GETTING MORE INFORMATION.

This means ASKING QUESTIONS, for increasing your information and clarifying your understanding.

By making sure you understand what the doctor has to say, you let them know that you are interested in listening. Also, you have increased your chances of the doctor's listening to you. We've all seen two people who have, instead of a conversation, two alternating monologues.

110

You can change the monologue pattern, however, by giving the doctor a chance to speak—and RISK being the listener! The information is important for you in order to digest instructions on prescriptions, dietary considerations, work habits, amount of sleep. The clearer your understanding, the better your chances for getting well.

Writing things down is essential. It is very difficult to remember a lot of new information, especially if it is technical or carries emotional content. We know one doctor physician who hands his patient a pad and pencil just as he begins to give his instructions. He wants to be sure the patient gets it right. He then reviews it to verify that what the patient wrote was what he said. Writing things down in the doctor's presence also convinces him you are really listening.

With listening skills, practice and a positive attitude, you can help your doctor recognize your life-threatening situation. You begin to take charge of your own recovery.

KEY WORDS

In order to take your notes more effectively and assure yourself that you are getting all the information, there are several additional listening techniques for you to try. The first is KEY WORDS.

Key words are words or phrases that appear to be stressed by the talker, are unusual or unknown to you, or are emotional or technical in nature. Key words need to be verified so that you're sure you understand them. If Dr Smith says, "Mary, you need to eat smaller meals more often during the day", there are several important key words to address.

The first is NEED. Why do you need to? What is the reason for not eating at regular meal times? The second is SMALLER. Well, how small? The third is MORE. Three more? Six more? It is critical to get ALL the information in order to understand thoroughly.

How do you use key words? ASK the speaker what they mean and how they affect you. "I don't understand. What do you mean by small?", "I'm confused. Why do I need to do this?"

In asking your questions, it is important to take responsibility for your own misunderstanding or confusion. "I don't understand", is easier for the other person to relate to than "You are not being clear". Emphasizing working together to get correct information helps you gain the support you so desperately need.

PARAPHRASING

The second technique is 'PARAPHRASING'. Paraphrasing is re-stating in your own words what you believe the other person said.

Saying something your way often helps you to understand it better. Deciding to paraphrase helps you focus your attention so that you can be on the lookout for key words. It also demonstrates your listening efforts.

An extra benefit is to give the speaker a chance to add or subtract from his or her statement, or to say it more specifically. Not all of us speak in perfectly edited sentences that contain our precise meaning!

With paraphrasing, you and the speaker become partners and team players, and establish a better appreciation of each other and the problem you are trying to solve.

For example, Dr Smith might say, "We are not sure how severe your Candida is. We'll have to run several more tests over the next two weeks. In the meantime, we want you to go on a special diet that is high in protein and low in carbohydrates. We also suggest that you exercise at least three times a week".

You might respond, "Let me make sure I understand: your diagnosis shows that I need more tests, a diet and special exercises. Is that correct?" Obviously, there is a great deal of specific information to learn, and the paraphrasing has given you a starting point.

From here, you can use your other skills such as 'key words', 'asking questions', and, of course, 'paraphrasing' in order to find out everything you need to know. Remember, get information. The more information you have, the fewer misunderstandings you will have to contend with. The net result is you get better faster.

ASSUMPTIONS

A third technique is 'checking your assumptions'. Historically, communication experts have told us not to 'assume'. However, we believe the assuming is not the problem; it is acting on our assumptions as though they were facts that gets us into trouble.

Assuming is a natural process. Where would we be if a scientist never made a hypothesis, which is just a sophisticated assumption?

How can we make assumptions work for us instead of against us? We can use our assumptions as a springboard to open up new and creative options for our current situations and problems, the way scientists examine a new theory. By checking and verifying our ideas, we can use them for a better understanding of the speaker and of ourselves.

'Checking out assumptions' is similar to paraphrasing—we are confirming parts of the speaker's conversation. We want to know what the speaker is really saying. We all have vivid imaginations and varied frames of reference, and can hear strikingly different meanings and possibilities within the same data.

Making assumptions can be great fun. The central ingredient, however, is allowing yourself the luxury to be wrong, silly, creative, maybe even a little off the wall. No great achievement, whether financial, scientific, or political, was successful without controversial ideas, mistakes and false starts. If you remember this, you may not worry about 'looking dumb'. You will be able to disclose and verify your assumptions—and get valuable information.

We would not have had the opportunity to write this chapter for Luc's book if we had not assumed that communication was important to helping Candida patients and that we might be able to be of assistance.

How do we use assumptions? When Dr Smith said, "We are not sure how severe your Candida is, we'll have to run several more tests", you can make a number of assumptions. You might feel that Dr Smith does not understand your case. You might believe that this process is never going to end. You can also feel that you are having to take time off from work for tests you don't think you need. The list can go on and on.

However, these assumptions are perfect grist for the mill in your ongoing dialogue with your doctor. If you do not clear these up, you run the risk of doing things wrong, doing too much, or undergoing unnecessary procedures.

These assumptions are SIGNALS to you to get more information. They are an opportunity to learn more about yourself and use your new information appropriately. This takes a bit of courage, however.

It takes courage and some diplomacy to let your doctor know if you feel he is not on track with you. You might start by saying, "Dr Smith, I think I've been a little unclear with you. First of all, I don't remember whether I told you I was already on a high protein, low carbohydrate diet and I'm exercising three times a week. So, I'm assuming I am not communicating properly. Let's see if there are other areas we need to review".

Another response might be, "Dr Smith, I feel that this therapy is going on forever. I just don't see any end in sight. And I'm not enthusiastic about all this new work", or, "Dr Smith, I can't see how I am going to be able to do everything you're recommending, and still work full time".

With these ideas or assumptions out in the open, both you and your doctor can begin to develop ALTERNATIVES. Working as a team, you can create a more structured and defined programme that is understandable and has an end in sight.

For example, you might devise your diet and exercise programme so that you have more time. It could become a family affair instead of your project exclusively. But, it will not get resolved unless it's brought out into the open with everyone cooperating.

The key to checking assumptions is being willing to say what's on your mind. Be sure to do this without accusing the other person of not listening, being unclear or manipulative.

Then, when you get home and begin to act on any new instructions, you won't find yourself saying, "Oops, is this what he really meant?" You'll feel better if you've said that earlier in the surgery. You'll have his corroboration and support right from the start. You both win. Together you can help each other create a mutually agreeable plan.

To review the Listening Techniques:
1. Identify 'key words or phrases' and ask questions to clarify them;
2. Paraphrase or feed back to the speaker in your own words what you feel they are saying;
3. Verify your assumptions no matter how unusual they might seem to be to you;
4. Take responsibility for what is going on with you. Let others know so that there is no confusion.

If, after you've tried all our techniques and you're still not getting the support and help that you need, it is time to consider a new doctor. However, please do not look at the time and energy you have spent as wasted. You have learned new ways to communicate, you have learned more about yourself and your illness, and you have a clearer understanding of what you need from your doctor.

Armed with this information, you can now embark on finding a doctor who can help. You have new skills and you can use them to make the most of your new doctor/patient relationship.

Remember, life is a creative process and your Candida is no exception. So take advantage of your information and your skills to get yourself well.

Assistance from Family and Friends

The major difference between working with family or friends and your doctor is that the doctor is there to work with you. It is a professional relationship in which you are to receive a service.

Your family and friends are not a service organization. They have their own lives and their own problems. To get their support and assistance requires consideration for their needs as well as yours. The first thing to realize is that it's very difficult for them to understand and appreciate a disease they've never had, can't see, and have never even heard of!

Second, if you're having a hard time expressing what you need or how you feel, they are having an equally difficult time understanding you. They want to help, but they just may not know how.

Tough Times

With any disease, there are a lot of difficult or tough times. These might include not feeling well enough to go to work, even though you have a special meeting that day. It might be not feeling up to going on a family outing that you, your spouse and children have planned for a long time. You might not be open to having sexual relations because you do not have the energy or you don't feel attractive.

In addition, we often have tough times that do not relate directly to our physical symptoms. These could be situations where we feel we don't have the skills to deal with a particular circumstance. Going to lunch with the boss and having to order a special meal, for instance, or having to tell a neighbour that his chemical spray is giving you a major allergy attack. This is especially true when these situations are completely new to you.

Needless to say, times like these can be frightening and stressful. "What will my boss think of me?" "My neighbour probably thinks I'm crazy", "My spouse will think I'm not in love anymore". All these can be typical reactions, and difficult for everyone involved.

But as the problem comes from within us, so does the solution. We need everyone's understanding and support, which we can get by listening to them, and helping them listen to us.

115

Helping people get ready to listen

We often assume that family and friends are available to us whenever we want to talk. Maybe familiarity allows us to take their attention for granted. We believe it is actually our responsibility to be sure friends and family are READY to help us.

The best and most direct way to find out is to ASK. You might say to your spouse, "I need to talk to you. When do you think we could have 15 to 20 minutes of uninterrupted time?" Or, "My allergies are just killing me. I think part of it is cigarette smoke. Could we have some time to ourselves to talk about it?"

By using the 'three sentence rule' (to recapitulate: main point first, clarify briefly, ask for feedback), you have let the other person know what you want to talk about. Make it clear that when they are READY, you would like their assistance. Finding out whether people are ready to talk is a good daily habit, not only for life threatening diseases. When making either a business or social telephone call, it is considerate to ask whether this is a convenient time to talk.

The same consideration holds true in dealing with your Candida. If you need a lift to the doctor, don't wait until the last minite to find out who is available. Please, ask for help in advance! People need the time and the energy to prepare— except, of course, in an emergency.

But an on-going situation, like Candida, is usually not an emergency. You have to manage and plan for it.

Does this sound like just plain common sense? Well, good communication is often just that—consideration and common sense.

To review: HELP others to be ready to listen to you:
1. Plan ahead, know what your needs are likely to be;
2. Let people know what you need to talk about;
3. Ask them when they have the time to discuss this and set aside the time.

Getting Help

Having set the stage for your meeting, you can now begin to communicate your situation. Here we go back to our four standbys: 'three sentence rule', 'key words', 'paraphrasing', and 'checking assumptions'.

Please consider, too, a wonderful aid that Nature has provided: your ability to modulate your voice. Tone of voice, like a smile, can go a long way toward producing a 'helping' atmosphere.

In a 'tough time' with your neighbour, a good place to start might be: "Harry, I need your help. I think the chemicals you're using on your lawn are affecting me. My allergies are so much worse since you started your weekly spraying. I was wondering if we could work something out together. What do you think?"

In getting help, it is important to remember that there are many possible solutions. Starting out with, "Harry, if you don't stop using those chemicals on your lawn, I'll sue you", may only get you a punch on the nose.

If you want HELP, this really means you want THEIR help . . . a plan they have worked on with you.

The next step is to GET INFORMATION. You might find out that Harry has finished the lawn spraying for this year. You might work out something for next spring. You might find out that Harry has been spraying in the afternoon when the wind is up. Maybe he could spray at night. There are many possible solutions. This is your chance to find them together.

OPTIONS

Between you, you can discuss possible options and discover a solution that can work for everybody. Here is where you use 'key words', 'paraphrasing', and 'assumptions'. With these tools, we can seek new information that can help solve the problem.

To review these listening techniques:
1. Identify 'key words or phrases' and ask questions to clarify them;
2. Paraphrase or feed back to the speaker, in your own words, what you feel he or she is saying;
3. Verify your assumptions no matter how unusual they might seem to be to you;
4. Take responsibility for your condition, and let others know about it so that they are less confused.

WORKING TOGETHER

Our students and clients have been amazed to discover that spending some extra time to explore options can produce quick results. A brainstorming session can offer a wealth of information. Here's how it works: you and your partners say whatever idea or plan comes into your heads, no matter how wild, innovative, outlandish it may be. No passing judgment—that comes later!

The first reaction many people have to this idea is that it will take too much time. It can—at first. But it saves time by preventing confusion and bad feelings later on. It often helps YOU feel better faster, and everyone else is happy to have played a part in your success.

An important benefit of this process is that it helps the listener appreciate your difficulties. It prevents a lecture or a long-winded dissertation, and becomes an idea they can relate to, within THEIR frame of reference. It is a process to discover something recognizable in THEIR background. It also helps remove the "If I haven't heard of it, it doesn't exist" attitude.

This takes a good deal of patience and understanding. But if you really need the person's help, it's worth it. Find out whether they have ever been so sick they could not function. Did they ever have something that was so hard to diagnose that no one would believe they were actually ill.

"Jean, if you have a moment, would you be interested in knowing what my problem is?" This may be one way to start the 'working together' process.

If they do show an interest, keep your explanation short and simple. You might say, "I got Candida from taking too many antibiotics when I was sick last summer. It upset the natural balance between the bacteria and yeast in my body. Have you ever taken medicine you thought was going to help but actually made you sicker?"

You might find out that when your neighbour was a child, they had a very serious illness that the doctors could not resolve. When the family moved to another town, the symptoms went away. The doctors there discovered that chemicals from a factory's smokestack had been causing the problem.

You might discover that there are many people with undiagnosed ailments—and that some of these ailments are actually Candida. Then you might be the one doing the helping.

Most people are ready, willing and able to lend a hand, especially if they are involved in DEVELOPING the solution.

To review: Working Together Better:

1. Maintain an atmosphere of HELPING and being willing to receive help;
2. Emphasize 'getting more information', ask clarifying questions;
3. Let the listeners in on the difficulties. Try to relate to something they may have experienced;

4. Take advantage and appreciate people's energy generated by their participation in the process of working out a solution—the successful culmination of brainstorming.

The Real World

Candida can turn normal every-day happenings into difficult problems, problems unique to Candidiasis. For example: You have been invited to the home of one of your spouse's friends for an elegant dinner party. You would love to go, but you are afraid of not being able to eat much of the food. You don't want to be embarrassed. But it is very important to your spouse for you both to be there.

What are your options? You could get sick the day of the dinner and not be able to go. You could bring your own food. You might eat first so that you nibble during the meal and avoid any yeast producing products.

But these ideas are yours alone. They don't consider your host and hostess. There might be some alternatives you might not have thought about. The only way to find out, however, is to ASK.

One possibility is to call your host or hostess and talk about it. "Mary, I was delighted to receive your invitation to dinner, but I have an eating problem. Do you have a few minutes to talk?" With that, you are on your way. "My doctor has me on a very strict diet. I would love to come but this diet is so limiting. Do you have any thoughts on how we could work this out?"

From there, you can begin to explore options. Your host or hostess might enjoy the challenge of creating a dish especially for you. Or, maybe the whole meal would be geared to the type of food you can eat—something new for everyone! If it is an informal get-together, you might bring along something for yourself that you and your host have worked out. The options are only limited by the interests and imaginations of the people working together.

To review: In order to be most effective in this type of situation:

1. Ask for HELP; let the person know your situation in advance;

2. Keep your communications short and informative, use the 'three sentence rule';

3. Maintain an attitude of HELPING;
4. Solicit your listener's ideas and support a team-work environment.

You can use these techniques in other family and friend situations. Most of the time they work, although they can sometimes be difficult to orchestrate. The most important thing is to RISK the possible difficulties of finding the help you need to get better—and enjoy yourself along the way.

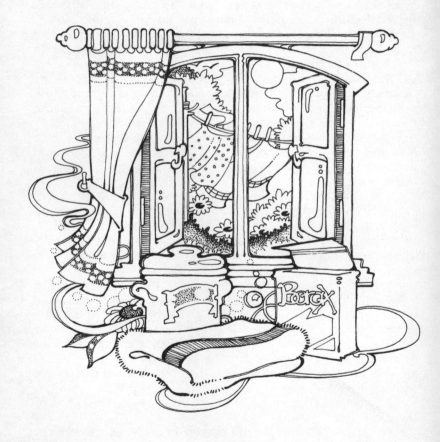

General Index

Index of Recipes

ABOUT THE AUTHOR

Luc De Schepper, M.D., Ph.D., C.A. is in private practice in Santa Monica, California. He is the author of *Acupuncture Within Everybody's Reach* (1980) and a medical textbook *Acupuncture for the Practitioner* (1985). He has a medical licence in Belgium, as well as in the states of California and Colorado. He obtained an acupuncture licence in Holland after completing a 3-year course at the Dutch Doctors' Acupuncture Association. In 1980 he obtained his Ph.D. in Acupuncture in Paris. He studied with masters such as Nogier, Borsarello, Mussat and Lebarbier and was a participant in the French National Congress of 1979–80–81 as well as in the World Congress in 1979 in Paris. After emigration to the U.S.A. in December 1981, he received his licence to practice acupuncture in California after passing the state examination. He was recently appointed Clinical Assistant Professor at UCLA Medical School, Pain Centre. He is fluent in four languages, English, French, Dutch and German. Dr. De Schepper is one of the most renowned lecturers in the field of Acupuncture and has lectured at Acupuncture schools and to licenced Acupuncturists in Europe and the U.S.A.